HEALTH REFORM FOR OUR TIME

DIET

BY

DESIGN

FRUITS
NUTS
AND
NATURAL
FOODS

**AN UP-TO-DATE
DIET AND HEALTH RESOURCE
COMPLETE WITH FRUIT AND RECIPE GUIDES**

Tyler J. Stanley

Drawings
Jeanette Stanley
Lewis Lavoie
Tyler J. Stanley

Cover Painting
Lewis Lavoie

Published by

TEACH Services, Inc.
254 Donovan Road
Brushton, New York 12916-9738

The author is not a medical practitioner and therefore does not diagnose diseases or prescribe the use of any of the information contained within this book. The reader is responsible for his or her own health, and any dietary or lifestyle changes that one makes (or persons that they have counseled after reading Diet by Design) are the sole responsibility of the individual (or individuals involved). If any of the information within this book is used without your health care provider's approval, the author or publisher is not responsible for any of the results.

Acknowledgments

The author is grateful to God for His mercy, grace, and guidance, and for impressing and inspiring several people to unselfishly assist in creating the work that now lies in your hands. May the Lord bless, according to His will, all who contributed.

Thanks to the staff at TEACH Services for their kindness, patience, and prayers.

CONTENTS

Introduction

As indicated by the title, the main purpose of this book is to encourage you to eat the diet originally given to man, and if you are like most people, this especially means eating more fruit. By thus doing, you will reap a broad spectrum of benefits. The physical gains are too numerous to mention and are interrelated with mental and spiritual development. Part 1 focuses on fruits as superior foods, outlines a basic dietary plan, discusses eating and lifestyle principles, and among other things, brings light to some of the controversial issues relating to food production. You will not be left stranded, not knowing how to put your newly acquired knowledge to use. In Part 2, the *Practical Fruit Guide*, you will learn everything needed to obtain the safest and most flavorful fruits. This guide is teeming with little-known shopping, storing, preparation, and health tips, as well as interesting facts. The illustrations add beauty and clarify each fruit's description. Part 3, the *Recipe Guide*, provides some excellent alternatives to many of the highly processed foods commonly eaten today, and will therefore help you to make a smooth transition into a natural, personalized dietary regime.

May this resource prove to be a blessing for all.

❏ It is true that people (due to varying circumstances) have different capacities to handle fruits. Experiment on yourself and eat larger quantities as your body permits (adjusts). Most can expect some initial eliminative symptoms. This is a good sign since it indicates that the body is discarding fat, diseased tissue, and various toxins.

Animal Testing

The author does not endorse animal testing; however, where appropriate, some animal studies have been described in this book. These have been included to expose the hazards that face people, rather than to support animal testing. Unquestionably, millions of animals are needlessly tortured and slaughtered every year in the name of science. By heeding the advice in the following pages, you can do your part (by eating and living naturally) to withdraw support from the industries who conduct animal testing. These industries include pesticide and drug manufacturers. Your responsibility is to grow as much produce as you can, to buy organically grown foods whenever possible (affordable), and to eat and live in a manner that allows your body to function within the established laws that govern all things.

Part 1

Rationale

Chapter 1

Character, Composition, and Benefits of Fruits with Comparisons to Refined Foods and Animal Products

Character

What Are Fruits?

There are differing opinions as to what makes a fruit, a fruit. Logically examined, it must be concluded that fruits are the edible portions of trees and woody plants, and that encase or contain seeds. Nuts are botanically classed as fruits but rightfully deserve their own category, perhaps "nut-fruits," because the edible parts are actually the seeds themselves. These delicious, nutrient-dense foods are discussed in various sections of this book.

Without question, fruits are the most aesthetically pleasing of all foods. Their visual appeal is delightful enough, yet they have been created with a wide variety of unique and wonderful aromas and tastes for us to enjoy.

Composition and Nutrients

Fruits are incredibly designed, possessing a perfect complement of sugars, organic acids (citric, malic, etc.), vitamins, minerals, enzymes, pigments, fiber, and starch. Everything is provided to enable the transformation from the immature stage until the fully colored, nutritionally complete, edible state. Enzymes trigger the conversion of starches to sugars, and generate softening and color changes. Sugars and organic acids impart the flavors. To ensure complete development, it is essential that those fruits that do not ripen further once picked (grapes, citrus, berries, etc.) be left until ready, and all others (pears, stone fruits, mangos, etc.) be harvested only after becoming fully mature.

Analyses of food composition tables clearly reveals that every nutrient known to be required by humans can be found in raw fruits, nuts, and seed-yielding plants—vitamins B_{12}, K, folacin, and others are synthesized by bacteria or contained in small quantities within a number of fruits and other plant foods.[1, 2] Be aware that nutrients are interrelated: for example, vitamin C, which is generously supplied in fruits, increases iron absorption. Fruits and nuts in the fresh raw state, are high in potassium and low in sodium, while processed and other undesirable foods have a reversed ratio. Common sense tells us that the potassium to sodium ratio in fruits and nuts is normal. One would have to eat approximately 500 pounds of grapefruit, 100 pounds of watermelon, 100 pounds of almonds, 35 pounds of dates, and 25 pounds of bananas—*all at the same meal* to equal the sodium in two bologna sandwiches![3] *The New England Journal of Medicine* reports that a high intake of potassium from food may protect against stroke related death.[4] Clearly, raw fruits are ideally suited for the human body—vegetables, sprouted or cooked grains and beans, tubers, and other unprocessed natural foods will be discussed later.

Organic vs. Inorganic, and Supplementation

Our focus thus far has been partially directed towards the adequacy of raw fruits, nuts and other plant-based foods in providing the vitamins and other nutrients required by the body. It is commonly believed that massive doses of vitamins and minerals are essential for health. In truth, we only need minute quantities of these *vital* "organic" substances. Using the maximum vitamin requirements, Dr. David Reuben has calculated one's *yearly* vitamin needs to be a quantitative amount so small that they would fit into a thimble![5] One thing we can be sure of is the fact that God has never made a mistake, and even with the condition of the environment today, if we farm (or shop) and eat wisely all the essential nutrients will be supplied from nature's bounty. Besides eating foods as they have been delivered-up in nature, we must avoid those substances that deplete existing stores, increase body needs, and interfere with normal absorption. The "robbers" and compromised foods include refined sugars and refined grains (white pastas, rice, breads, sugar, etc.), animal products, cooked foods (depending on the type), toxic substances such as alcohol, tobacco, drugs, caffeine (coffee, tea, chocolate, soda pop, etc.), *and even supplements*. We never have to worry about overdosing on vitamins as contained in unrefined natural foods because our bodies simply convert or absorb what we need and excrete the excess. This does not give one a license to overeat, because overeating places a heavy burden on the entire body, especially the kidneys, liver, pancreas, adrenals, and heart.

Note that some people have seriously damaged their ability to utilize nutrients and must faithfully incorporate and adhere to all the proper dietary and lifestyle requirements in order to realize positive results. A fast or series of fasts may also be required. Consult someone who is experienced in these matters.

Many less-desirable foods are enriched and fortified with vitamins and minerals, which brings us to the point where we must make a distinction between God-created and man-made nutrients.

Friends, only plants have the ability to take inorganic (non-organic) nutrient matter from the soil and convert it into the organic substances needed by man. To eat rocks (or drink mineral water) hardly seems like a logical way to obtain minerals. Just look at the inside of a kettle or water distiller and then imagine the damage that inorganic mineral matter could be doing to your blood vessels and joints. Inorganic vitamins can also be harmful, and even deadly. Non-organic supplements (vitamin, mineral, etc. preparations) simply cannot be substituted for the originals. Some supplements have actually been shown to cause deficiencies.[6] For example, megadoses of vitamin C, B_1 (thiamine), or multivitamin preparations could cause a B_{12} deficiency.[7] Other negative effects from taking supplements include stone formations, gastrointestinal problems, arthritis, diabetes, heart disease, blood vessel damage; kidney, liver, and glandular problems; blindness, infertility, fetal death or deformities, and cancer, to name a few.[8, 9, 10] Let us examine several supplements and expose some of the hazards.

Iron is required in very small amounts because the body recycles most of its supplies from the red blood cells before they are discarded. Only in rare instances can one use more than that provided in whole natural foods. Taking inorganic iron pills can cause hemochromatosis, a nasty disease where iron builds up to the point of causing diabetes, impotence, heart failure, and eventually liver cancer![11]

Vitamin A supplements pose a substantial threat, especially for pregnant women. A recent study (Rothman et al) published in *The New England Journal of Medicine* (and discussed later in the *Lancet*) proved without a shadow of doubt that vitamin A (retinol) supplementation by pregnant mothers causes birth defects.[12] Rothman says, "our data indicate a large increase in the prevalence of birth defects at doses that are easily achieved from supplements now available."[13] This is particularly disturbing considering the fact that many people megadose, with hopes of obtaining greater "benefits."

Beta carotene, as found in orange and yellow fruits and vegetables, cannot cause birth defects because the body converts what it needs into vitamin A, and excretes or stores the excess.[14]

Vitamin D, taken unnaturally as inorganic supplements, can cause kidney stones[15] (calcium is drawn from the bones and teeth and deposited as stones). Vitamin D is produced by the body when the eyes and skin are exposed to the sun's rays; and therefore, it has been coined the "sunshine vitamin." Exposure to artificial lights is harmful.

Vitamin E supplements are a major hazard to those with high blood pressure or rheumatic heart disease, and taking them could quickly result in death![16]

Vitamin C & E: One study found that those who took 1000 IU of Vitamin E and 2000 mg of vitamin C daily, had twice the death rate of the group who did not take supplements.[17]

Folic acid supplements could be hazardous by suppressing symptoms of pernicious anemia, which when left to run its course, causes paralysis.[18]

Calcium supplements have been positively associated with osteoporosis and vascular disease.[19]

We could discuss others, but sufficient evidence has been provided to enable one to see that our nutrients should (under normal circumstances) come from raw and other unprocessed foods.

Inorganic or synthetic supplements are, for the most part, stimulants as can be verified by anyone who immediately and completely discontinues their use. Feelings of weakness, headaches, dizziness, and uneasiness are among the possible symptoms.

But what about nutrients derived from "natural sources?" Well, that is a broad term and could mean almost anything depending upon the nutrient being discussed and the producer making the claim. Vitamins, minerals, phytochemicals, enzymes, etc. made (dried) from *organic food sources* appear to be safe (*if* 100 percent pure) and *could* be beneficial in cases of deficiency; however, the author's experience indicates that people simply need to make the positive (and necessary) dietary changes and to live in harmony with the other laws of health as described in a subsequent chapter—this process becomes enjoyable when one perseveres.

It is true (though extremely rare) that one could still become deficient in some nutrients even while eating a diet that includes raw fruits and vegetables. For example, iodine deficiency could occur if the soil from which one's foods were grown was deficient in this nutrient. Such a case can easily be prevented by obtaining produce from different locales or by using seaweed as an occasional seasoning agent. Seaweeds happen to be the highest known food sources for iodine, and also contain B_{12}—a vitamin which has been needlessly used to strike fear into vegetarians. Swiss chard, turnip greens, summer squash, mustard greens, watermelon, cucumber, asparagus, kale, turnips, okra, blueberries, rutabagas, peanuts, strawberries, sweet peppers, and many other fruits and vegetables normally contain iodine.

As you read this book it will become apparent that fruits and nuts are well-endowed with organic nutrients. Listed under each fruit's nutrient heading (in the *Fruit Guide*) are some of the more significant vitamins and minerals contained in each, with hopes to dispel any fears, substantiate the information in this section, and for interest sake. Do not become obsessed with nutrients because it is unlikely that you will ever have to worry about them again if you eat plenty of raw foods—as stated, with rare exceptions.

Sugars: Fruits vs. Refined

Fruits take priority over all other foods because they not only furnish our vitamin and mineral needs, but our greatest requirement from foods—*calories*, in the form of readily available sugars. Dried fruits are a super-concentrated source.

It is not surprising to hear people say that they are always craving sweets and highly sugared junk foods, because it's only natural to desire sugars since they appeal to the most pleasurable taste sense—*sweet*, and allow for harmonious functioning of our physiological apparatus. Glucose is the fuel that our bodies run on, whether we supply it directly (and primarily) from fruits (various unprocessed sugars) as God intended, or abnormally stress the organism to derive it from substandard and detrimental foods. The brain runs on glucose! Natural sugars as supplied in fruits are accompanied with all the other necessary nutrients required for proper metabolism. *When fruit sugars are not provided, one turns to counterfeit alternatives.*

❏   Note that grains, legumes, and nuts supply glucose at a slower rate (beneficial for many); however, since these foods are acid-forming, whenever possible, they should constitute the lesser portion of the diet. Non-acidic vegetables that are good sources of glucose (tubers, squash, etc.) may be successfully eaten in greater quantities when necessary. See *Acid-Base Balance* and *The Optimal Diet*.

The ease and efficiency with which fruits are digested is unsurpassed by any other food. They are gently and quickly transported from the stomach to the intestine for further processing. Included are generous amounts of fiber and water needed for gradual sugar absorption and to carry wastes from the system.

In contrast, sucrose and other refined sugars (the counterfeits) contain 0 vitamins, 0 enzymes, 0 trace elements, 0 protein, 0 fat, and 0 fiber, along with a minute amount of impure iron,[20] and *all the calories*. Truly, sucrose and like sugars, along with their pharmaceutical effects, should be classified as drugs. This becomes evident when we consider the physiological damage that results when one avoids fruits and yet attempts to obtain an energy boost (a "high") by eating refined sugars. Refined sugars (and refined grains) are highly concentrated and rapidly absorbed, and this greatly stresses the endocrine glands (pancreas etc.) and creates an abnormal, fluctuating blood sugar state, which in turn is responsible for the "sugar high." This elevated state is quickly followed by a miserable letdown.

To illustrate the concentrated nature of refined foods: Refined sugars and grains are about 99 percent concentrate as compared to 15 to 20 percent for dried fruits,[21] which in of themselves provide more glucose than some people can handle. One would have to chew the sugar out of twelve feet of sugar cane to equal four teaspoons of white sugar![22]

Other hazards of refined sugars include diabetes, hypoglycemia, severe immune system depression, dental caries, osteoporosis, obesity, heart disease, cancer, gastritis, constipation, thiamine depletion, depression, nervous disorders, hyperactivity, an increased craving for alcohol, and criminal behavior.[23, 24, 25, 26] Refined sugars also increase blood fat levels, which in turn cause red blood cells to clump together. Sluggishness, poor functioning of the entire body, and increased risk of heart and vessel diseases are the disastrous results.[27, 28]

Sugars and the Immune System
White blood cells lose their ability to engulf and destroy germs (phagocytosis) in correspondence to the amount of refined sugar consumed. An experiment conducted by Dr. Ralph Steinman produced significant results. Volunteers were tested over 20 minute periods. When the people did not consume refined

sugar, their white cells could destroy 14 germs. With just 6 teaspoons of sugar, 10 germs could be destroyed. After 12 teaspoons, only 5 germs could be abolished. With 18 teaspoons, 2 germs, and after 24 teaspoons, just 1 germ![29], [30] Sanchez and his colleagues had similar results, and found that the undesirable effects from just one sugar feeding lasted up to *five hours*.[31] The relevance of these findings is greatly enhanced when one considers that a single can of pop, a chocolate milkshake, or a cinnamon bun *each* contain 10 teaspoons of refined sugar. With all the hidden sugars in today's processed foods, many people actually consume over 150 teaspoons per day! No wonder immune system diseases are so prevalent in westernized societies.

Among the refined sugars are white, brown, turbinado, and fructose sugars, corn and maple syrups, and molasses.

Honey: Fit for Food?
The Bible states instances of honey being used as a food source (likely in small amounts as a sweetener) and therefore its use cannot be entirely condemned; however, like many other foods being produced today, honey is becoming unsafe and one would need to buy from a reputable source. There are far better sweeteners such as dates or date sugar, but if you prefer honey then buy it directly from a bee-keeper who does not use chemicals during production or collection time.

Botulism poisoning (often lethal), especially in infants, is another possible hazard of honey.[32]

Perhaps it will help some readers to know that one cancer patient who was doing well on an all raw food diet was given honey to increase his weight—and he died.[33]

One must also be aware that honey possesses an undesirable sugar ratio. Fruits contain 5 to 8 percent fructose, while honey has 40 to 52 percent[34], [35]

Finally, some honey is pasteurized (cooked). Cooking deranges and destroys nutrients, thus making honey a liability to the acid-base balance of the body—see *Raw vs. Cooked* and *Acid-Base Balance*.

Taking all into account, whenever possible, other sweeteners (such as dates or date sugar) are recommended in place of honey.

Artificial Sweeteners: Saccharin, Aspartame, and Cyclamates
Cyclamates, now banned, are known carcinogens. Saccharin is associated with bladder cancer in humans,[36] and causes kidney damage and birth defects in animals.[37] Aspartame is known to induce headaches and seizures, and causes brain tumors in animals.[38], [39] One study with human volunteers showed that the calories "saved" on an aspartame-sweetened diet were quickly compensated for by the consumption of more food.[40] Aspartame also

increases one's appetite, especially for sugars[41] and fats[42] —one of a dieter's worst enemies!

❏   *Undoubtedly, fresh and dried fruits are the sweets that have been provided for people.*

Sugars, Diet, and Dental Health

Dental diseases fall into three main categories: caries, periodontal diseases, and erosion. Let us examine these and their relationship to diet, giving particular attention to refined sugars (and honey), fruits, and juices.

Dr. H. T. Knighton demonstrated (human test subjects) that eating whole apples eliminated 96.5 percent of mouth bacteria (averages given) and whole oranges abolished 95 percent, while tooth-brushing and a water rinse only removed 64 percent. Pre-cut oranges registered at 56.9 percent.[43] He correctly concluded that chewing increased salivary flow, and swallowing completed the removal process. This destroys some common assumptions, but does eliminating bacteria prevent tooth decay? Dr. Howe found that bacteria had no affect on the teeth of monkeys as long as their diet was natural.[44] Even though monkeys are animals and we are human beings, this study is relevant because natural laws are in force for all of creation. Incidentally, monkeys eat a large portion of whole, fresh fruits.

When Howe fed different animals refined sugars and grains, meat, eggs, pasteurized milk, and coffee—no different from the atrocious diet that many people eat—they developed rickets, scurvy, decayed teeth, and other diseases.[45] He correctly determined that refined sugars and other harmful substances (taken alone and especially together) perverted the overall metabolism and brought disease to the entire body, including the teeth. High-protein or vitamin C-deficient diets were particularly harmful. Orange juice was successfully used as a restorative in the "scurvy diet."

Dr. Shelton, on reviewing the works of Dr. Howe and others, stated that anything that disrupts calcium metabolism destroys the teeth and bones. Also, that when proper conditions are reinstated to a diseased body, that it can restore some or all of the normal functioning of the teeth, but not structural damage. Additionally, his research indicates that teeth develop caries from the *inside*, and these become visibly evident when the enamel is broken through.[46] Studies conducted at the Loma Linda University also indicate that tooth decay begins on the inside.[47] Incredibly, this is contrary to what was, and is, commonly taught and believed. Truly, diet and living practices are the underlying factors in the causation of dental caries, and this is where the emphasis must be placed.

The health of Eskimo peoples has been thoroughly studied, comparing pre-white contact with dental and other disease rates. Archeologists obtained

246 skeletal samples of Eskimos who did not have contact with whites, and found the carie rate to be very low. The results were attributed to traditional diets free from refined sugars, food additives, and starches.[48] This is not to say that a high-fat diet is healthy; in fact, the Eskimos have always been short-lived peoples. The lack of caries in those on a traditional Eskimo diet may be partially attributable to abnormally large amounts of chewing (food, leather, etc.), which stimulated salivary flow and the metabolic processes within the teeth (as directed by the brain). Archeological studies of other peoples have produced similar results: very few, if any caries, and enamel about twice as thick as those living in the westernized societies of today.[49]

Another study on Eskimos showed their average sugar intake in 1959 to be 26 pounds, and just eight years later, to have reached an astounding 104.2 pounds![50] Those with the highest intakes of refined sugars had mouths full of carious teeth. Diabetes, gallbladder disease, and abnormal growth patterns became the norm. Obviously, a high-fat diet combined with refined sugars equals disease.

Refined sugars [likely honey as well] have been shown to slow down the fluid circulation within the tiny canals of the teeth (fluid moves outward from the pulp and through the enamel), drastically increasing the incidence of caries and preventing proper mineralization.[51, 52] Complete omittance of refined sugars is necessary if one desires proper mineralization of the teeth. The decrease in fluid circulation caused by refined sugars (and probably other substances) creates the opportunity for bacteria to play a secondary role. Also, be aware that refined sugars and honey encourage the formation of plaque.[53]

Erosion has been positively associated with the intake of soft drinks, coffee, and other undesirable beverages,[54] as well as refined sugars.[55]

Some studies have shown fruits to be slightly erosive, although the entire diet, maturity of the fruits, and one's living practices need to be considered in these cases. Animals who were fed a diet of grapefruit, guava, Java plum, mango, and pineapple, experienced little or no enamel erosion, but feeding them the juices of these same fruits caused significant erosion.[56]

Linkosalo studied a large, easily divisible population group and determined that the salivary composition and its flow rate or buffering capacity were factors in preventing dental erosion. Elevated levels of salivary amylase, magnesium, and protein, along with a high flow rate, corresponded with less erosion.[57] Whole fruits definitely increase salivary flow as was shown by Knighton, while juices do not stimulate salivary secretions adequately and promote overeating—a habit that disrupts metabolism and blood chemistry, particularly when cooked foods are overeaten (easily done). Linkosalo did make positive correlations between juice drinking and erosion, but the erosions were not severe;[58] conversely, Howe experienced positive results with orange juice feeding. As reported in the *International Journal of*

Pediatric Dentistry, children who consumed the most drinks (in general) and fruit drinks had the highest rates of erosion, yet whole fruits "did not reveal statistically significant differences."[59] *The Journal of the Canadian Dental Association* reports that processed fruit juices have a pH below the "critical dissolving pH of enamel," and are therefore "potentially hazardous to teeth."[60]

Daily juice drinking is contraindicated when fresh fruits can be obtained, to prevent erosion and overeating, and to encourage mastication (increases flow rate)—especially important since many foods today are prepared in a manner that simply requires swallowing. Only fresh-squeezed fruit juices are suitable because they have not been cooked, and do not contain refined sugars and other harmful additives. Commercially processed juices have been cooked (pasteurized), and this not only alters their pH, but makes them poor sources of nutrients—both of these effects disrupt the acid-base balance (see *Acid-Base Balance* for more). Processed juices also contain higher levels of pesticides.

Realistically, fruit acids merit attention because many fruits are harvested prematurely. Unconverted fruit acids do have an erosive effect on the teeth, with unripe acid fruits being the worst. One would be wise to avoid unripe fruits that do not ripen further once harvested, and to wait for all other types to reach the height of perfection before consuming.

Periodontal health is encouraged by daily consumption of whole raw fruits, nuts, and vegetables because these foods provide the necessary stimulation, in addition to the perfect complement of nutrients. Fruits supply the vitamin C naturally needed to make pyorrhea a disease of the past. Diets based on refined sugars and refined grains, or proteins, are responsible for mouth and bone diseases because they disrupt the acid-base balance and are inadequate in nutrients, especially vitamin C.

Raw nuts should not be underestimated in value when striving for dental and overall health, due to their outstanding distribution of mineral matter, fatty acids, and protein—all undamaged by cooking. Nuts are considered to be "anti-tooth decay" foods.

Cleaning food particles and residues from the teeth (even fruits, particularly dried ones) with a soft brush, water, and floss is apparently a beneficial precaution to prevent plaque build-up and bacterial action, but does not, and cannot take the place of a healthful diet.

Considering the evidence, it must be concluded that any diet or living practice (stress, negative emotions, poor eating mechanics or atmosphere) that creates impure blood and perverts metabolism will lay the foundation for dental and other diseases. Obviously, mastication is important to encourage salivary flow, as well as intestinal secretions and many other metabolic processes. A diet abundantly supplied with whole, fully mature fresh fruits, with the addition of raw nuts, seeds, and vegetable matter, encourages proper eating mechanics and provides the nutrients required for superior health of the teeth, gums, and entire body.

Mothers must be aware that the prenatal development of teeth and skeletal structures is vital—the child does not have a second chance! A nutrient-rich diet and freedom from circumstances that trigger stress responses are required for the mother and the developing child. Artificially fed infants develop high rates of decayed teeth[61] —breast feeding has many benefits that cannot be provided any other way.

Refined Foods—Additional Comments
The information given to this point clearly shows that refined foods (sugars, grains. etc.) have a destructive influence on the body. They most assuredly "sow the seeds" of ill health. These seeds sprout overnight as manifested in acute diseases, and as the dosing continues, chronic diseases develop. Make no mistake about it, refined foods pervert the appetite and sense of taste, and lay the foundation for disease. People become addicted to the products that contain these health destroying substances and cannot appreciate the delicious flavors of natural foods—even fruits in severe cases. Those who have been blessed with children bear the weighty responsibility of providing foods that will allow them to grow and function optimally.

Protein, Fats, and Fiber—Fruits vs. Animal Products

Most fruits are naturally low in fat and protein, the two dietary components that are routinely eaten to excess in westernized countries. Both protein and fat needs can be amply met from raw fruits and nuts alone when adequate calories are consumed.

Protein
True protein requirements have been estimated to be as low 10 grams per day, and most unbiased researchers set needs at about 30 grams per day.[62, 63, 64] This figure is but *one-half* of the recommended daily allowance (RDA), which undeniably caters to the meat, egg, and dairy industries. Many in North America consume over 100 grams of protein per day, primarily from animal products. Significantly, upon digestion, flesh foods impart a large amount of nitrogenous wastes, including ammonia, urea, and creatinine. These substances excessively tax the liver and kidneys[65]—in truth, the blood becomes poisoned so the entire body suffers. Furthermore, animal products putrefy in the digestive tract, and this causes exceedingly toxic by-products to be formed and disrupts and perverts one's natural intestinal flora, setting the stage for colon cancer. Conversely, in the natural state, fruits are clean-burning, relatively toxin-free foods!

Fats

Fruits that are high in fat and protein, oily fruits (avocados, coconuts, and olives), and nuts and seeds, definitely have their place in a natural diet, and for superior results, these should be the only high fat and protein sources. They are cholesterol-free and provide an excellent complement of usable fatty acids, vitamins, minerals, and protein (amino acids); however, to obtain these nutrients they must be eaten raw and in moderation.

Many people are afraid to eat these delicious and very satisfying high-fat fruits, fearing that the fat will go straight to their thighs or waistline. This is an incorrect assumption. Avocados for example, contain 1.7 calories per gram as compared to 7.2 calories per gram for butter or mayonnaise.[66] The calories in avocados can be easily utilized, and the fat is largely monounsaturated. Monounsaturated fat discourages high cholesterol levels. Nut and seed fats are the most beneficial fats because they are comprised of high percentages of linoleic and linolenic acids, both of which have a marked effect in reducing one's chance of dying from coronary heart disease.[67]

But what about coconuts; don't they contain a lot of saturated fat? Yes, coconuts are comprised of about 92 percent saturated fat. However, *The American Journal of Clinical Nutrition* reports that pure vegetarians who consumed up to 25 percent of their *fat calories* from coconut, did not have greatly elevated levels of cholesterol, and their levels were substantially lower than those compared who used animal fats.[68] Another significant study was conducted on members of the Philippine armed forces. Though they commonly used coconut products, they did not have elevated levels of serum cholesterol.[69] Carefully note that both the pure vegetarians and the Philippine military personnel consumed low percentages of total dietary fat, and also obtained regular exercise.

Once again, the main danger lies with animal products (flesh, eggs, cheese, butter, milk, and all other dairy products) because they contain large amounts of saturated fat and cholesterol. Foods in the plant kingdom do not contain cholesterol. Organ meats and eggs top all other foods for cholesterol content. Saturated animal fats represent the main causative factor in the development of arteriosclerosis, which in turn results in high blood pressure, heart attacks, and strokes. Butter is a stimulant[70] that, like all other animal fats, hinders digestion and clogs the blood. Cheese (high in protein and fat) is mucus-forming (as are all dairy products) and putrefies in the digestive tract. Most commercially sold cheeses contain rennet, a substance taken from the stomach of a newborn calf or hog.[71]

Unquestionably, animal fats can have disastrous effects on the body; however, any diet that is comprised of too much fat will result in disease. Fat can be consumed to excess in three ways: by eating animal products, using oils and margarines, and finally (but less likely), by eating too many natural foods that are high in fat.

Saturated vegetable fats (solid at room temperature) such as margarines are also unfit for the human consumption. Margarines contain a host of additives, preservatives, and waste products.

Vegetable oils have received a lot of good press, but close examination reveals a different picture. To begin with, extracting the oil from whole foods eliminates the fiber. Secondly, almost all oils (excluding cold-pressed) have been subjected to high temperatures, and if they haven't, most consumers are likely to do so anyway. Cooking the oil destroys or deranges the vitamins and minerals, makes them largely indigestible, and causes free radicals and carcinogens to form. Finally, oils are extremely concentrated. It takes *fifteen* ears of corn to produce just one tablespoon of oil![72] In light of the facts, oils are best used in very small amounts; or better yet, eliminated altogether when adequate portions of raw high-fat foods are included in the diet—avocados, nuts, seeds, olives, and so forth. Actually, all foods contain fats but simply in varying amounts.

Fiber

Everyone is well aware of the importance of fiber in the prevention of developing diseases (notably bowel cancers, diverticulosis, and heart disease)—so where can you get your fiber? *All* animal products are fiberless, while all fruits and other plant foods are fiber-rich. Animal products putrefy (rot) in the digestive tract and destroy natural bacterial flora, while at the same time, encourage the development of abnormal bacterial cultures that play a role in causing cancer. Conversely, fruits are soft, easily and quickly transported through the intestine, develop and support normal bacterial flora, and are packaged with a superior complement of nutrients. Dried fruits are particularly high in fiber, with figs being a better source than bran flakes. Nuts also contain generous amounts of fiber, as do vegetables, whole grains, and legumes.

Factory Farmed Animals and Disease Transmission

The fact that high-fat and protein diets lead to disease should encourage one to adopt a vegetarian diet, but the quality of animal products and the methods used in their production deserves even greater consideration. To begin with, the treatment of factory farmed animals is truly inhumane. Overcrowding and brutality is commonplace, and the suffering can be seen, smelled, and heard. A host of chemicals are fed or injected into the animals including antibiotics, hormones, sulfa drugs, tranquilizers, pesticides, and arsenic derivatives. They are also fed the following "materials": feather, blood, bone and fish-meals; animal fat, buttermilk and whey powders, yeasts and by-products from the brewing industry, *sewage*, cement dust, chalk, limestone, dolomite, and cardboard.[73] Other meals contain sawdust saturated with ammonia, and newspapers containing toxic inks.[74] The obvious result of feeding animals poisons, wastes, and foods contrary to their natural dietary—is disease.

We too become diseased when toxins or unnatural foods are introduced into our systems. Drugs, prescription and non-prescription, are outright poisons that have no place in the human body. Drugs merely suppress symptoms and build chronic disease (see Appendix)—extreme health emergencies such as accidents or surgery may require temporary treatment. Additional offending substances include perfumes, colognes, cosmetics, pore-clogging deodorants, and other toiletries. Avoid these, and use the money saved to purchase those foods that naturally keep the body clean—fresh raw fruits and vegetables (see *Cleanliness* for more).

The entire scope of drugs, other hazardous chemicals, and the diseases (including cancer) contained within factory farmed animals are passed on to humans through the consumption of their flesh, milk, and eggs! This translates to cancers, birth defects, mutations, and many other diseases in humans.[75, 76, 77, 78, 79, 80, 81, 82] In 1975 (things have gotten much worse since), one study found 75 percent of supermarket samples of cow's milk, and 75 percent of egg samples to contain the leukemia (cancer) virus. By 1985, nearly 100 percent of the eggs tested, or the hens they came from, had the cancer virus.[83] The animals themselves are often riddled with tumors, and those which are visible are simply cut off. Cancer is definitely transferred from animal products to humans, and amongst the scientific information that supports this fact: the highest rates of cancer belong to those who produce dairy products and eggs.[84] This is but a small part of a very dangerous and disgusting picture as you will soon read.

Beware!

It is also common practice to feed livestock carcass meal, a feed that contains the burnt remains of diseased animals, and obviously—*their feces*. One farmer says that 14 percent of animal feed in the United States is processed animal remains.[85] This senseless feeding practice is the one responsible for Bovine Spongiform Encephalopathy (BSE, 'Mad Cow Disease') in Europe which has a possible link to Creutzfeldt-Jakob disease (CJD) in humans—people are dying from CJD. Prions (infectious proteins that are not destroyed by high temperatures) are suspected to cause these diseases because they lodge in, and infect brain tissue—dementia results. Are North Americans safe? Apparently not: in 1985, an encephalopathy outbreak on a mink farm was the result of feeding them the remains of diseased cows.[86] Logically, the only sure way of prevention is total abstinence from flesh foods, as well as commercially sold eggs and dairy products.

Now that you know the etiology of this lethal form of dementia in relation to factory farmed animals, it should be obvious that all types of natural scavengers should be avoided at all costs. Nature's waste disposal system includes pigs, all shellfish and scaleless and finless fish, birds of prey, and every other abominable creature that feeds on dead, diseased, and poisonous animals. Scavengers have an increased threat of carrying potentially lethal poisons, as well as some of the more nasty bacterial, larval, and viral diseases.

Evidently, from the information presented thus far, it can be reasonably concluded that in a situation where a cow or chicken is fed blood, bone, fat, or flesh from swine, that the pig would become part of the cow or chicken (or their by-products), along with any diseases that it was carrying.

Bacterial, Larval, and Viral Diseases

Do not overlook the fact that only animal products are responsible for E-coli, salmonella, campylobacter, trichinosis, and a throng of other infections with bacterial, larval, and viral origins. Let us briefly discuss a couple of these avoidable problems.

E-coli has been in the forefront in the past several years. What is it, or what are they? E-coli are natural intestinal bacteria, but one animal strain, O157:H7, is hazardous and often fatal to humans. E-coli ends up in hamburger and other "edible" animal meats when they come in contact with *feces* during slaughter—a common occurrence! In 1993, undercooked hamburger from a chain of fast-food restaurants was proven responsible for over 500 culture-confirmed cases, including the deaths of four children.[87] Some of the infants and children who died did not even eat the meat, but came in contact with counters, loving hands, or feces from infected children.

Trichinosis is a relatively common disease (in varying degrees) that develops from the ingestion of trichina worms. These worms are largely present in pork products, but may be found in beef and other flesh foods. The worms may not be killed by heat because they are encysted in calcified cysts, and once inside the human body, each female can produce up to 1500 living larvae![88] The larvae grow before becoming enclosed in cysts which then calcify and can remain in the human body for years.[89] Symptoms from infections include intestinal disturbances, abdominal pain; painful, swollen muscles; fever, and difficulty in breathing and swallowing. Death can occur in severe infections.[90]

In light of the facts presented thus far (also see chapters three and four), the reader should seriously consider abstaining from all flesh foods, eggs, and dairy products. Obviously, these foods would have to be replaced with an abundance of raw fruits and vegetables, and lesser amounts of raw nuts and seeds and other unrefined plant foods—feasible to most in North America who live and shop smartly.

Enzymes

Enzymes are necessary for food metabolism (among other processes). Raw fruits and other plant foods not only encourage proper enzymatic production within the gastrointestinal tract, but are themselves abundantly supplied with these vital catalysts. All cooked and processed foods lack enzymes, and this places an enormous strain on the body as it struggles to compensate for the difference. Cooked proteins have enzyme-resistant links form between amino acids.[91] A denatured (cooked) protein cannot be restored: for example, a coagulated egg. Most enzymes cease to function at around 131°F (55°C)—body temperature is approximately 98°F (37°C).

Water

Fresh fruits contain high percentages of the purest solvent available: distilled water. We are living in a polluted world, and therefore it is necessary to take extraordinary measures (obtaining distilled drinking water) to provide our bodies with the pure water they so desperately need. Among the many forms of water purification, distillation is the most effective, so it makes even more sense to supply a large percentage (at times all) of your body's water requirements naturally—with fruits! Those who eat larger quantities of fruit, particularly melons (when in season), will have little desire to take water or any other beverages. Hot weather could cause the need for extra water; however, thirst may not be the most accurate guide for some people. One should consume enough water (through foods and/or distilled drinking water) to keep the urine pale yellow or clear.

The generous quantities of water in fruits, along with the readily available glucose, aids the body (directed by the brain) in determining a normal satiation point, thereby signaling one when to stop eating. With adequate water intake, constipation could be a soon forgotten problem, and desires to drink harmful beverages will be diminished or disappear altogether.

Besides fruits and vegetables, most foods are practically waterless. Store-bought drinks are thought to be an excellent source for pure water, but in reality they are poor sources at best, and most are outright harmful. Even mineral and spring waters are unsatisfactory due to the inorganic minerals and wastes they contain. Rainwater is impure due to the filth in the air. Let us examine some of the water dangers in processed foods. To do this, we simply need to analyze tap water. Tap water contains thousands of contaminants including heavy metals, pesticides (all farming poisons), PCB's, dioxin, hospital and nuclear waste, and raw sewage! Over 700 chemicals have been identified in U.S. drinking water, including 129 that the Environmental Protection Agency calls "dangerous."[92] The chlorine and fluoride added to our water supplies—to "purify" them, and to make us "healthy"—are *highly poisonous*. Studies link chlorine to a number of cancers, especially those of the bladder, colon, and pancreas.[93, 94, 95, 96, 97, 98, 99, 100, 101] Research verifies that fluoride causes an increase in cancer (fatal and otherwise),[102, 103, 104, 105, 106] osteoporosis (bones and teeth),[107, 108, 109] birth defects,[110] and a decrease in birth rates.[111] The latest research shows a positive correlation between fluoride intake and brain damage, as well as lowered intelligence.[112, 113] Need it be said that children are small people who are developing brains and nervous systems! Do not forget that toothpastes are laced with fluoride.

Obviously, the importance in supplying the body with pure distilled water cannot be overemphasized. One is better off spending more money on fresh fruits than on distilled water; however, due to temperature changes and the variety of fruits available, everyone should have a non-food source of distilled water. Buying a water distiller is an excellent health investment that will quickly pay for itself. You cannot put a price on health once it is lost.

Acid-Base Balance

Our bodies must maintain a delicate balance, and the foods we eat play a key role in developing and sustaining healthy blood, fluids, and tissues. Actually, we have three masterfully designed regulating systems: acid-base buffers, the kidneys, and the respiratory system; all work to keep the blood and lymph within the narrow parameters that support health (pH of 7.35 to 7.45). However, disobedience to dietary laws will necessarily override the ability of these systems to cope. The result: acidosis or a lowering of alkalinity—note that the blood and lymph never really become acidic, for this would bring a speedy death.[114]

The degree of alkalinity or acidity of a solution is indicated by a numerical value and the symbol "pH" (water, 7.0 pH is neutral), and the acidity or alkalinity of the solution is determined by the hydrogen ion (H+) concentration.

When a food (or substance) is ingested and metabolized it either leaves an alkaline or acid ash, denoting the predominating minerals that remain after it has been used by the body. Minerals that have a high hydrogen ion concentration are called acid-forming minerals, while those that have a low hydrogen ion concentration are called alkaline-forming minerals. To elaborate, those minerals that release hydrogen ions are termed acid-forming, while those that accept hydrogen ions are alkaline-forming. Sulphur, phosphorous, and chlorine are the acid-forming elements, while potassium, sodium, calcium, magnesium, and iron comprise the alkaline-forming elements.

The nature of a food prior to its consumption generally does not reflect its nature after it has been metabolized. For example, before an orange is eaten it is classed as an acid fruit, but the ash left after metabolism is decidedly alkaline, and thus we refer to the orange an alkaline-forming food. Fresh fruits, with few exceptions (plums, olives, carob, and some berries) leave an alkaline ash, as do vegetables, while animal products, grains, most legumes, nuts (excluding the almond, chestnut, and coconut), and seeds leave an acid ash. The significance lies in the fact that the body maintains a ratio of approximately 80 percent alkalis and 20 percent acids, and will do everything possible to keep this balance intact.

Acid-base buffers (buffer salts) are one of the methods used to control alkalinity. The body recognizes free acids as being harmful and quickly binds them with alkalis, rendering them harmless. Specifically applying this to dietary intake, when acid-forming foods are eaten their acids must be bound by alkaline minerals (salts). Ideally, these alkalis are supplied by alkaline-forming foods that have been eaten at the same meal or from reserve supplies within the blood. However, when acid-forming foods are eaten to excess, and reserve supplies have been depleted, then the condition of acidosis exists (lowered blood alkalinity). At this point, the body has no choice but to draw alkalis (bases) from the bones, teeth, and other tissues, thus setting the stage for osteoporosis, dental caries, and other diseases.

Potential symptoms of acidosis include mild or chronic fatigue, nervousness, headache, sleeplessness, acid stomach, acid perspiration, colds, or an ill disposition.[115] Chronic abuse damages the kidneys and other organs.

Obviously, one must guard against eating too many acid-forming foods, and it would be better to eat fewer because acids are also contained within alkaline-forming foods, simply in smaller proportions.

Not surprisingly, flesh foods are exceedingly acidic and can quickly deplete the alkali reserves normally contained within the blood, before gradually sapping those of the bones, teeth, and other tissues. Flesh foods leave a residue containing sulphuric, phosphoric, and uric acids, all of which heavily stress a number of organs and the regulating systems of the body, notably the kidneys, lungs, and liver. As previously stated, the lungs and kidneys are also important in regulating the alkalinity of the body fluids. The lungs control the amount of carbon dioxide in the system—carbon dioxide increases acidity—and the kidneys excrete either acids or alkalis in the urine. The first step in improving acid-base balance: eliminate flesh foods.

In addition to flesh, all other animal products are highly acidic as well as unsafe and should be avoided. In descending order, the acid-forming foods which *are* deemed appropriate include acid-forming fresh fruits, raw nuts and seeds, mature corn, whole grains, and legumes.

Briefly, we shall discuss how refined and other denatured foods affect the acid-alkali balance, with hopes that the reader will be motivated to totally eliminate these substances from their diet. It is necessary to understand that in order to metabolize and utilize any food, a specific compilation of vitamins and minerals must be supplied, preferably and primarily from the food itself—as our Creator intended. From previous discussions on refined and processed foods, you already know that they are lacking or almost totally void of vitamins and minerals. Now, when vitamins and minerals are not adequately prepackaged within the food itself, the body has no choice but to draw from the reserves that freely circulate in the blood and lymph—if any are available. Assuming that the reserves are inadequate (due to poor habits) the body has no other alternative but to access the tissues, primarily the bones and teeth, thus beginning the downward trend toward osteoporosis and dental caries. The hazards of refined foods and supplements were discussed more fully earlier in the chapter.

Some of the other dietary abominations that disrupt the acid-base balance and poison the body include coffee, tea, chocolate, cocao, and products that contain vinegar.[116] Vinegar, as you are probably aware, contains acetic acid. Taking this acid into the body creates an emergency in a hurry, and for self-preservation, calcium and other bases are leached from the blood, bones, teeth, and other tissues. Vinegar is extremely damaging to the red blood cells and could cause anemia.[117]

Medical preparations that contain acids are also highly hazardous to the body and markedly disrupt the acid-base balance. Acetylsalicylic acid is one such drug.[118]

Looking at the opposite end of the scale, alkalosis is also a variance from the norm. Alkalosis can occur due to kidney or lung damage, from over-breathing, or from the use of antacids.[119] Antacids (including baking soda) should never enter the human body.

To conclude, it is essential that the preponderance of the diet be comprised of alkaline-forming foods, and that every food that is palatable when raw should be consumed as such. It should be evident that our bodies have been wonderfully designed and function as a whole, and that we simply need to live within the health-sustaining boundaries that have been established, nothing more and nothing less.

Chapter 2

Buying and Eating Fruits For Nourishment

Raw vs. Cooked

Fresh raw fruits represent the ideal, and most people living in North America can obtain them if so desired.

Cooking is Harmful—Four Prominent Reasons

1. Cooking destroys or denatures the vitamins and other nutrients in fruits, and for this reason, avoid cooked fruits whenever possible.

2. Cooked fruits, being poor and unbalanced sources of nutrients, disrupt the acid-base balance, and thus sap the body of vitamin and mineral reserves. In contrast, raw fruits possess all the nutrients required for normal metabolism and impart an alkaline ash, thus building up vitamin and mineral reserves.

3. Mutagens develop when a food is cooked, with meats (pork, beef, poultry, seafood, etc.) and other animal products (eggs, milk, cheese, yogurt, ice cream, butter, etc.) being by far the worst offenders.[120]

4. Free radicals (damaging compounds with unpaired electrons[121]) are formed when foods are cooked. Cooked oils, flesh foods, and other animal products are exceedingly hazardous in this regard.

Cooking foods that do not need to be cooked can only lead to less than optimal health. Obviously, some foods must be cooked in order to be edible: various tubers, winter squash, and mature grains. Consuming cooked foods alone cannot provide the materials required to attain or sustain vibrant health. This applies to people as well as animals.

The most famous animal experiment proving this point was conducted by Dr. Pottenger. He divided cats into groups and observed the effects that raw and cooked foods had on the animals. The cats who were fed raw foods thrived; while those receiving cooked food developed a number of diseases including bone deformities, paralysis, cyanosis of the liver and kidneys, degeneration of the nervous system and brain, enlarged colon, and sterility by the second or third generation![122]

Truly, the human body has been wonderfully designed and can withstand a lot of abuse, including an adulterated diet; however, natural laws cannot be transgressed without penalty, and the sure result is disease and early demise. The atrocious state of health of peoples (on the whole) in westernized societies is evidence enough to prove this point. This is not to suggest that cooked foods should be eliminated from one's diet, but they should not comprise the majority of the food consumed. As stated earlier, cooked fats and animal foods represent the greatest hazard—by far. Most plant foods that require cooking are nourishing and satisfying, especially during the winter months.

Canned Fruits—Store-bought
Store-bought canned fruits (and vegetables) have been fragmented and cooked, thus destroying most of the vitamins and altering or abolishing the other nutrients. Canned fruits often contain refined sugars, and carry with them the dangers of fluoride, heavy metals, and high levels of pesticides (especially tomatoes). If you decide to eat canned fruits, then be sure that they have been packed in their own juice and are free from sugar and other undesirable preservatives.

Frozen Concentrate, Bottled, and Carton Juices
Frozen concentrate, as well as carton and bottled juices have been pasteurized (cooked), and contain high levels of pesticides due to improper preparation of the fruit and the concentrated nature of the finished product. Commercially sold juices have been made with tap or filtered water rather than pure distilled water. Using tap water in cooking or food preparation greatly increases one's intake of poisons, including fluoride—for fluoride dangers refer to the section on water.

Whole vs. Fragmented

It is always in your best interest to consume fruits (or any food that can be eaten raw) in the whole state, thereby minimizing oxidation, and subsequent destruction of nutrients. Oxidation rapidly occurs when the fruit's flesh is exposed to air. Any process that creates this condition is moving away from the ideal. For example, cutting cantaloupe into wedges an hour before consuming it causes free radicals to form, and depletes stores of the antioxidants beta carotene and vitamin C. The trouble is twofold since free radicals (compounds that accelerate the aging process) are in direct opposition to antioxidants ("anti-aging" nutrients such as vitamins A, C, E, and selenium). Melons deteriorate extremely fast so it makes sense to buy them whole, and to cut them immediately before serving, avoiding leftovers if possible (see *Watermelon* in the *Fruit Guide* as an exception). If you find it more appealing to eat melon in wedges or balls, do so, but remember that it would be highly advantageous to do the preparations immediately before serving.

Some will find the shakes, salad dressings, and other recipes in Part 3 to be nice additions to their dietary regime; however, these items should not be eaten to the exclusion of whole fruits. Obviously, juices are far less desirable due to their extensive exposure to oxygen. Avoid all juices that have not been freshly extracted, and keep these to a minimum (For an in depth explanation, see *Sugars, Diet, and Dental Health*).

Blended fruits are preferable to juices, but should also be minimized unless dental problems prevent thorough chewing.

Immature and Overripe Fruits

Unfortunately, many fruits are harvested prematurely. The result: underdeveloped, poorly flavored, lower nutrient-value fruits. Study the *Fruit Guide* to learn how to pick mature fruits.

The unconverted acids within immature fruits can cause tooth enamel erosion—for an in depth explanation, see *Sugars, Diet, and Dental Health*.

Fruits that have been harvested too early prove to be a terrible waste, and do not possess the essential complement of nutrients. They lack flavor, will never develop properly, and are generally destined for the compost bin. Hard, unripe, decaying cantaloupes are a prime example. Pears and other fruits that ripen best off the tree are discussed in Part 2.

Overripe specimens are worse than useless because the process of fermentation has already begun. Fermenting fruits contain poisonous alcohols (similar to those people buy), which once taken into the body, annihilate brain cells—lost forever! *Never* consume overripe fruits. A sloshy honeydew is a perfect illustration. Fermenting fruits emit an alcoholic odor and have an off taste in relation to the degree of spoilage. Tips for spotting fermented fruits are provided throughout this book.

Chapter 3

Diet, Health and Longevity, Weight Loss, and Personal Performance

After reading the previous chapters it should be evident that an abundance of raw fruits and moderate amounts of raw nuts and seeds (barring allergy) should be included in everyone's diet—a vegetarian diet. In this section we will expound on this further, linking the optimal diet to health, weight loss, longevity, and physical and mental performance.

A Case For Vegetarianism (elaborating on Chapter 1)

Pure vegetarian diets (no animal products but an abundance of fruits) have been shown to decrease one's risk of developing cancers, heart disease, strokes, and osteoporosis. Hypoglycemia and Type 2 diabetes can improve or be rectified, and Type 1 diabetes is easier to handle. High blood pressure may be lowered. This all equates to an increased life span with superior endurance as compared to non-vegetarians![123]

An extensive study on one easily-segmented population group in California found that persons who did not use animal products [pure vegetarians] lived the longest by a wide margin, and with far fewer diseases![124, 125] They had 86 percent fewer heart attacks than the general population, while the second section of the control group, lacto-ovo vegetarians [people who use milk (dairy) and eggs], had 61 percent less.[126] The people eating a pure vegetarian diet consumed higher percentages of fruits and nuts than both the lacto-ovo vegetarians, and the third section of the control group: the omnivores [people who use flesh, dairy, and eggs]. The pure vegetarians had substantially lower levels of serum cholesterol than the lacto-ovo vegetarians and the omnivores.[127]

From the facts presented thus far, we can hereby conclude that man possesses an innate drive to desire more raw natural foods, and in proper proportions, as one's health improves. Also, that diets high in protein and fat accelerate growth and cause early maturation, which in turn leads to disease and a shortened life span.

The "China Study" (1983–91), examined the diets and diseases of Chinese peoples in various regions of China. Comparing the Chinese statistics with American disease rates and the Standard American Diet (SAD) proved most revealing. The Chinese eat diets low in fat and cholesterol but high in fiber and vitamin C, with almost all protein being derived from plant sources, while the American diet is opposite in every respect. Cancer and osteoporosis are rare in China but major problems in America. Only one percent of the Chinese population dies of coronary artery disease, as compared to 50 percent in the United States![128] One might think that Chinese people are going hungry, but think again; they actually consume more food than Americans—superior food. Dr. Colin Campbell, one of the researchers involved in the China Study, says that animal protein is probably a more significant factor in cancer and other diseases than fat.[129]

One final example should suffice: the Hunzas of Pakistan. The Hunzas are one of the longest-lived peoples in the world and possess incredible endurance and strength. So what is their secret? Simply this: they eat a natural diet, work vigorously in the fresh air every day, and the worries of life are kept to a minimum. Their diet consists primarily of fresh and dried apricots, with lesser amounts of peaches, apples, cherries, watermelons, grapes, pears, and mulberries, as well as raw nuts, vegetables, grains, and beans. Approximately 80 percent of the their diet is eaten in the raw state—even the beans are sprouted and eaten raw.[130] This raw-to-cooked-food ratio is ideal for most people, taking into account the cooler temperatures during the winter months.

❑ Sadly, in recent years, the poisons of westernized countries (junk foods, TV, etc.) have begun to invade and destroy the Hunzakuts.

The Optimal Diet

The optimal diet is one that supplies the body with all of its nutrient needs, appeals to the senses, and allows one to function at peak levels, both mentally and physically. In short, a diet based on fresh and dried fruits, with moderate amounts of raw nuts and seeds, and generous portions of leafy greens and a variety of other vegetables. Lesser amounts of whole grains and legumes (sprouted whenever possible) are valuable additions, especially in the winter. By and large, cooked grains and legumes are acid-forming, as are nuts and seeds, and acid-forming foods should never comprise more than twenty percent of the diet—be watchful. The evidence given thus far indicates that a fruit-based diet is the one originally given and best suited for man rather than one based on grains, animal products, legumes, nuts, or seeds. Those who have difficulties that prevent them from eating large quantities of fruits should eat more tubers (potatoes, yams, rutabagas, etc.), squash, other starchy and non-starchy vegetables, and sprouts because they are alkaline-forming (with few exceptions).

During the summer, when a large variety of peak-season domestic fruits are available, one can (and does) live beautifully on raw fruits, nuts, and vegetables alone—fresh fruits taking priority. Of course, if you want to base your diet on these wonderful foods you must be a wise shopper and purchase bulk quantities, paying particular attention to those items that are on sale. Better yet, cooperate with God in growing at least some of your own foods, thereby eliminating full dependence on industry, and partaking in the many benefits of gardening. For those on a small budget it is doubly important to buy fresh (and dried) fruits and vegetables rather than refined and canned foods, since processed foods are not only nutritionally corrupt—but expensive. Nut milks can be made for less money than cow milk! Finally, we can conclude that the optimal summer diet is the ideal year-round diet wherever the weather permits.

During the winter more dried fruits and oily fruits such as avocados should be added to the diet. In cooler weather, when more heat must be generated, cooked foods can be handled much more efficiently. Cooked grains, legumes, and other starches (winter squash, yams, pumpkins, potatoes, etc.) are best accompanied by plenty of raw foods: fruits or vegetables (especially leafy greens), according to correct food combining principles. Remember, summer or winter, acid-forming foods should never comprise more than twenty percent of the diet.

According to one study, cooked foods may not be required. As reported in the *Journal of the American Dietetic Association*, Jaffa studied a "fruitarian" family (including two children) whose diet was almost entirely made up of *uncooked* fresh and dried fruits, and nuts. He found the children to be in excellent health but under the average height and weight of "normal" children.[131] He concluded that this was partially due to heredity. Truly, "normal" is probably abnormal since most children are raised on meats, eggs, cheeses, butter, milk, and other dairy products—foods that cause abnormally rapid growth (see *Children*). If not for any other reason, the diet cited in this study should be encouraging to those who are unable to digest or obtain a large variety of foods, showing that the quality is the most important factor to consider.

It should comfort the reader to know that researchers have found pure vegetarian diets to help both children and adults to maintain or achieve desirable blood lipid levels.[132]

❑   The optimal diet should be quick to prepare so that more time may be spent with family and in productive work and study—fruits are *suncooked* and ready to enjoy!

Personal Performance

Who likes to be mentally dull, incoherent and lacking in energy? Suffice it to say that a fruit-based vegetarian diet creates the healthiest blood and therefore allows the brain and entire body to function efficiently and effectively. Fruits must be given the highest priority since they are clean-burning and require but little energy to digest. Your reward: increased energy levels.

Children

Is a pure vegetarian diet suitable for children? Being the diet given at creation, certainly it is, and children who are raised as vegetarians develop few (if any) of the common childhood diseases. Infants need milk from their own mothers, who themselves should be eating a vegetarian diet and living according to the laws of health. By analyzing the table below, we can obtain a better understanding of the importance of breast-feeding.

Average Chemical Composition Percent

Type of Milk	Fat	Protein	Carbo-hydrates	Minerals	Days to double birth-weight
Human	3.95	1.60	6.25	0.45	190
Cow's	3.70	3.55	4.88	0.71	47
Goat's	4.50	4.30	4.40	0.80	19

* Chart compiled from information contained in The Science and Fine Art of Food and Nutrition and the Hygienic Care of Children.

It can be seen that cow milk contains more than twice as much protein as human milk, and that calves double their birth-weight in less than one-fourth the time of a child. Also, that cow milk does not contain the percentage of carbohydrates required by an infant. Human milk is perfectly designed to nourish the slow, steady growth of the body, and significant growth of the brain. The human brain is greater in size at birth than that of any animal, and also develops quicker.[133] The most important differences are not distinguishable from the chart: Cow milk contains too much casein, is insufficient in milk sugar and albumen, and is poorly digested by the human infant.[134] Significantly, mother's milk contains lecithin bodies which are essential for brain development, and for the first few days after birth, a special chemically adapted secretion called colostrum is afforded to the child.[135] Colostrum contains antibodies and proteins that strengthen the immune system, and also has laxative properties.[136] Breast milk is non-allergenic, available, economical, rarely causes diarrhea or vomiting, and it is less likely that the baby will be overfed[137]—a habit that will be very difficult to break.

Quoting from *The Science and Fine Art of Food and Nutrition*, "In view of the superior fitness of mother's milk to nourish the human brain, it comes as no surprise to learn that mentally, breast-fed children are brighter and indefinitely superior to bottle-fed children. Bottle-fed babies are more neurotic, have more of the 'diseases of childhood,' and a higher death-rate. It has been repeatedly shown that breast-fed babies are physically and mentally superior to bottle-fed babies. Except for height, bottle-fed babies rank lowest in all physical traits measured."[138]

Referring back to the table, you will notice that goat's milk is even less suitable for an infant than cow's milk.

According to Drs. John Tilden and Herbert Shelton, mother's milk and *freshly-squeezed* fruit juices should be the only foods given to children until the age of two (soaked and strained dried fruits included).[139] This makes sense since one needs a set of teeth to be able to chew foods. Regular eating times should be established from the first feeding. Dr. Shelton advises mothers to wean infants gradually on a wide variety of fresh fruits, vegetables, and raw nuts (but not peanuts). Regarding starches, he says, "Before the teeth are fully developed the saliva of the infant contains a mere trace of ptyalin, the digestive ferment or enzyme that converts starch into sugar. There is just enough of this ptyalin present in the saliva to convert milk sugar into dextrose. It is this almost total absence of starch-splitting enzymes from the digestive juices of the infant that accounts for the great amount of digestive disorders which result from feeding starch foods to infants. When starch digestion is impossible, starch fermentation is inevitable. This poisons the baby."[140]

During physical growth, including the development of the brain and nervous system, it is vital that children are provided with the proper nourishment. Their requirements are easily supplied through the natural desire for more food (plant foods). Children need adequate portions of fruits and moderate amounts of nuts or seeds every day (barring nut allergies). Bananas, dried fruits, avocados, and olives (if obtained from a safe source) should be made available, letting the child enjoy those foods that are preferred from that which the parents themselves have been provided with—from nature's bounty as opposed to junk foods. Foods that the child deems repulsive should not be forced upon them.

Children should be lovingly, patiently taught the essentials of healthful living, including the importance of proper dietary principles. They should be on a regular eating schedule and adhere to the food combining and eating principles outlined in chapters seven and eight (along with the parents). They should be encouraged to be temperate, yet should not be deprived as to be ill-nourished.

Pregnant Women

Pregnant women require more food, including larger quantities of dried and fresh fruits, avocados, olives, raw nuts or seeds, leafy greens and other vegetables, and a variety of other unrefined natural foods. During pregnancy and lactation, it is even more important that the mother adheres to a strict vegetarian dietary regime, practicing temperance, yet being sure that both herself and the child are adequately nourished.

Diabetics

Diabetics can and do eat large portions of fruits without difficulties. In fact, diabetes is rare among peoples who live primarily on fruits, vegetables, and starches.[141] Diabetics need to greatly restrict their fat intake and eat unprocessed, natural foods. Experiments have shown that diets high in fat, and low in carbohydrates and fiber are largely responsible for diabetes.[142] Dr. John McDougall is in full agreement with these findings, encourages diabetics to eat fruits, and stresses the importance of eating foods in a raw, natural state—this cannot be overemphasized. Obesity also plays an important role in causing diabetes because fat causes the tissue cells to become less sensitive to insulin.[143] Evidently, the two major factors that diabetics (everyone) must seriously consider are diet and exercise. Dr. McDougall reports that up to 75 percent of Type 2 (adult-onset) diabetics can eliminate their need for insulin shortly after making the outlined dietary change; and Type 1 (juvenile) diabetics can usually reduce their dependence on the drug.

Significantly, *The New England Journal of Medicine* reported that juvenile diabetes was strongly linked to the protein within cow milk.[144]

Major Dietary Changes Or a Transitional Approach?

Transitional dietary reform will prove to be the most successful course for most people; however, make no delay in giving up flesh foods, condiments and other substances that contain vinegar, fermented foods, irritating spices, refined grain and sugar products, highly saturated fats, and outright poisons such as caffeine (coffee, tea, sodas, chocolate, etc.), alcohol, and drugs that are not needed to support life. The recipes in Part 3 are especially helpful for those who use a transitional approach.

Others will feel compelled to quickly eliminate all that is unnatural and highly processed, knowing that major dietary changes *may* cause some people to feel worse initially. Temporary symptoms should not cause alarm, because it simply means that the body is detoxifying. For the most part, detoxification occurs when fat cells are broken down, thus causing stored toxins (poisons) to be released into the bloodstream. This is a beneficial process because poisonous waste matter and fatty and diseased tissue is rapidly discarded, and this results in weight loss and greatly improved health. Those who do not want to lose weight can expect weight loss, but this can be regained in healthy muscle mass after the body rids itself of the unwanted materials, and when more concentrated foods are eaten in conjunction with vigorous physical work.

The catabolism (breakdown and detoxification) phase may (or may not) produce symptoms such as headaches, weakness, cold and flu discomforts, and general malaise. Those who experience such symptoms should be patient and simply let the body do its cleansing work without suppressing the symptoms (by taking non-lifesupporting prescription or non-prescription drugs etc.)—do not interfere by putting in what the body is trying to throw off (see Appendix). Before long, fruits (and all foods that used to taste bland—even plain romaine lettuce) will taste better than you could ever imagine, energy levels will greatly increase, and most importantly, your thought processes will be acute, providing the capability for constructive development of the mind—character development. Obviously, one cannot expect to fully reverse twenty or thirty years of destructive living in a few days or weeks, but huge strides can be made, and with perseverance, substantial health gains (noticeable and unnoticeable) will be achieved. To minimize the effects of detoxification use a transitional approach, and for genuine and lasting results stick to a program that includes the lifestyle practices discussed later in this chapter.

Your health is your responsibility! You have the freedom to eat and live in the manner in which you choose. Adopting a program that allows you to function efficiently, both mentally and physically, is the goal.

❑   People on drugs, or those who have taken large doses of drugs in the past, may experience additional discomforts or adverse affects when making a major dietary change. Special care may be required.

Weight Loss, Exercise and Other Lifestyle Factors

Obviously, diet is an important factor in a healthy lifestyle, but there are other vital elements that must be provided in order to achieve genuine, long-lasting results—in truth, we do not make ourselves healthy, but sick; health is natural, although not "normal."

The human body has been designed to move. People who enjoy daily outdoor exercise (nature walks, gardening, etc.), in conjunction with eating a natural diet, experience steady, safe, and permanent weight loss (normalization, until the body decides on the ideal weight) as long as they continue with this healthy, vibrant way of living. Recent research backs up this common-sense approach (including sticking with the program), crediting a low-fat diet and exercise with raising the percentage of fat (stored fat) in the fuel mix and improving the metabolic profile.[145] It has been shown that those who exercise have elevated basal metabolic rates even while sleeping—almost six percent higher![146] Exercise should not be overly strenuous, especially for those who have been eating a high fat diet, are sedentary or under a lot of stress, or have a family history of cardiovascular disease.

Studies show that endurance is substantially improved when one eats a high carbohydrate diet. One Swedish study centered on nine athletes whose physical endurance was measured while on stationary bicycles. They were fed three diets during the testing, which produced the following results: A diet high in protein and fat equated to a miserable average of 57 minutes riding time at the preset work load. A varied diet doubled their performance. Finally, a high carbohydrate diet produced superior results with an average of 167 minutes riding time![147] The significance lies in the fact that fruits are the finest high carbohydrate foods. Dried fruits are super-concentrated sources.

Thus far we have elaborated on two major essentials of health, a natural diet and exercise. If you are wise enough to get outdoor exercise, then that gives you a third—*sunshine*, and if you avoid traffic and other pollution sources, a fourth—*fresh air*. Other essentials include *pure water* (see *Water*), *cleanliness* (inside and out), *mental and spiritual soundness and growth, adequate rest and sleep*, and most importantly, *love*. Every one of these factors is vitally important, and one's health will suffer to the degree that any of these are lacking.

Fresh Air

As one exhales, carbon dioxide is expelled. This cellular waste product is being disposed of for a reason: it prevents oxygen from reaching the cells of the body! Therefore, obviously, it is vital that we have a continual source of oxygen-laden air or we will be doing nothing more than breathing in our own filth. A constant supply is needed—24 hours per day and 365 days per year! Anything short of this is contrary to the creative design of the body. Obviously, the poisons within tobacco smoke and vehicle exhaust are highly destructive and cancer-causing.

Sleep

The most beneficial sleep is obtained prior to midnight. One should adhere to a program of "early-to-bed and early-to-rise." Of course, windows should be open to provide fresh air.

Cleanliness

Inside, by eating a diet based on raw fruits, and by following the *Tips for Healthy Eating and Food Combining* in chapters seven and eight. Outside, by washing the body daily (twice if needed) and by wearing clean clothing. Actually, internal and external cleanliness are directly related to one another because the toxicity and degree of poisons on one's skin reflect the toxicity and degree of poisons in the body, and in turn, if the wastes on the skin and clothing are not removed, they will be re-absorbed into the system.

Sunshine

Avoid extended periods of direct exposure from 10:00 a.m. to 4:30 p.m. during the summer months, and year-round if you live in a hot climate. Vitamin D, necessary for proper calcium metabolism, is produced as a result of exposure to the sunshine, and therefore, it is essential to obtain direct exposure during the non-peak (safest) hours of the day. Being fat-soluble, vitamin D can be stored for future use (during the winter months when less sunshine can be obtained), so get adequate amounts during the summer. The face should receive most of the exposure, and this is the case when proper dress is worn.

Mental and Spiritual Soundness and Growth

Is realized through study of the Scriptures, prayer, the sharing of one's faith, and most importantly, the grace and love of God; and is significantly enhanced when one works with the Great Physician to establish proper dietary and other living habits.

Love

"Behold the Lamb of God, which taketh away the sin of the world" as He hangs beaten, bruised, and bleeding on the cross of Calvary—bearing the sins of mankind!

Chapter 4

Obtaining Safe Food

Avoiding safe food issues would be unrealistic, so let us investigate, keeping a positive outlook. The facts and suggestions that follow will expose most of the dangers and give you the knowledge necessary to protect yourself, your family, and anyone with an open ear. Refer to the section entitled *What You Can Do To Greatly Reduce Your Intake Of Pesticides* until the suggestions given have been incorporated into your food preparation regime. If the subject of pesticides bothers you, please do not ignore this entire chapter, but rather follow the recommendation above and read *Suggestions for Obtaining Organically Grown Fruits*.

It is not the author's intent to cause fear, but merely to provide answers for those that have concerns regarding safe food issues. Rather than being a stumblingblock, it is my prayer that the information in this chapter will help someone to overcome a physical ailment.

We have much to be thankful for, and by eating the diet that has been designed for us, our meals, with a blessing from above, can be eaten with assurance and cheerfulness.

Pesticides vs. Organic AgriculturePesticides

Chemicals are toxic, potentially lethal substances that were originally developed for use during W.W.II. At the close of the war they were incorporated into agriculture and household products, and the sad results are a witness to all—chemical-free foods had been grown, provided, since creation nearly 6000 years before. Chemicals have lasting, hazardous effects on our soils, water (even rainwater), and the very air we breathe. Those chemicals used in the production and treatment of our foods fall under the term "pesticides," and include insecticides, herbicides, fungicides, and many others. Make no mistake about it: almost all are used to kill—most veterinary drugs have been classed separately, are used in conjunction with pesticides, and pose equal or greater risks.

Of the 1000 pesticides registered worldwide (more than 100,000 formulations[148]), well over 300 are used in North America, totaling 2.6 billion plus pounds per year in the United States alone.[149] With this enormous, ever-increasing arsenal, bugs, weeds, and fungi should be non-existent. This is not the case however; pests are developing resistance and crop losses are increasing. Twice the number of insects developed resistance to pesticides during a ten year span from 1970 to 1980.[150] Over 500 insect species are resistant to pesticides today, as compared to seven in the 1940's.[151] Do pesticides increase crop yields? Absolutely not. Pesticide use increased tenfold from the 1940's to the 70's, yet crop losses to insects doubled![152]

In 1995 alone, almost 29 billion dollars (U.S.) were spent on pesticides throughout the world.[153] The real cost however, is the irreversible damage done to humans, animals, and the environment—who dares to put a price on this!

Effects on Humans

Pesticides are responsible for cancers, liver and kidney diseases, nervous system and brain damage, birth defects, skin diseases, and every disorder related to the immune system. Cancers alone have shown a marked increase since the introduction of pesticides (and related chemicals) in the late 1930's.[154] From 1950 to 1990, cancer incidence rose nearly 50 percent,[155] and according to the American Cancer Society, the incidence of cancer in the United States is now 1 out of every 2.5 persons, and increasing.[156] It is estimated that 1,359,150 new cancer cases will be recorded in the United States for 1996.[157]

Children and farm workers are the most vulnerable. Children eat more food and weigh considerably less, and therefore receive a greatly increased intake of pesticides as compared to adults, and at a time when they are developing brains, nervous systems, organs—bodies![158] Furthermore, the "acceptable daily intakes" (ADI's) for pesticides in food are set for the average adult, and only take into account the particular pesticide in question and not the hundreds that can be consumed every day. Know that these chemicals are tested separately, and not in the combinations that end up being consumed. This most certainly creates the reality of unforeseen chemical unions and increased toxicities. Children also eat a larger percentage of foods that contain high levels of pesticides. The offending substances include milk, all other animal products, store-bought juices, and other processed fruits and vegetables. The Natural Resources Defense Council (NRDC) concluded that children receive four times the exposure (as compared to adults) to eight extensively used carcinogenic pesticides in food.[159] The National Cancer Institute found that childhood leukemia increased up to sevenfold when garden, lawn, and household pesticides were used.[160] Childhood brain cancer has been definitely linked to garden, lawn, and home pesticide use.[161]

Farm workers receive the most direct exposure because they breathe and have extensive skin contact with enormous amounts of pesticides every day. The World Health Organization estimates that 25 million farm workers in developing countries are poisoned every year,[162] and of these, over 20,000 die.[163] Approximately 300,000 farm workers in the United States alone are adversely affected by pesticides every year.[164] Farm workers have an increased chance of developing eleven different cancers.[165] Extensive and ongoing skin, lung, gastrointestinal, and neurological diseases are the norm.

Food

Without question, flesh and other animal products contain the highest levels of pesticides, however, we shall focus on produce first.

Undoubtedly, there are unacceptable levels of pesticides on many of the fruits and vegetables in the supermarkets—anything above zero. Strawberries, peppers, cherries, seedless grapes, and tomatoes are a few of the worst offenders but there are problems with most.[166] Sadly, it has been estimated that up to 80 percent of the pesticides used on food crops are applied simply to increase the eye appeal of the finished product,[167]—so don't always reach for that "perfect" fruit. Unfortunately, most of the chemicals are at least partially systemic, meaning that they become inherent within the cellular structures of the flesh, and therefore can only be washed off to the degree that the residues remain on the skin. Waxed fruits even prevent these from being washed off, and waxes frequently contain fungicides or absorb those that may be applied after the produce has been waxed.[168] Waxes may be derived from animal products,[169] or produced synthetically using the very same ingredients in car waxes.[170] Waxes, being a post-storage treatment, obviously do not extend the storage life of fruits and vegetables but are simply applied for aesthetic reasons. Those fruits that possess thick, inedible skins are far more desirable because the parts consumed are free from the direct chemical onslaught. Bananas, melons, citrus fruits, and mangos belong in this category.

Imports generally contain the highest levels of pesticides because they are always treated during transport and storage. Imports could easily contain double the pesticide levels, including chemicals already banned in North

America—like DDT![171, 172, 173] It is true that many carcinogenic chemicals are exported from the United States every year, only to result in having the poisoned food brought back into the country.[174, 175] Estimates indicate that 75 percent of the pesticides used in Third World countries are banned in the United States.[176] Considering local food supplies, know that DDT stays in the environment a long, long time, and accumulates in animal products, as reflected in a study by the Council on Environmental Quality that found meat and dairy products to account for 95 percent of the average person's intake of DDT.[177]

Take Heart, There's Hope!

One study focusing on people over 65 found that those who consumed large amounts of vitamin A (beta carotene) and C-rich fruits and vegetables [probably all non-organically grown] had one-third the mortality rate from cancer as compared to those who ate small portions of these foods.[178]

Studies with other population groups have produced similar results.[179] These results can be attributed to many factors including an increased intake of fiber, vitamin C, and beta carotene (from the foods), as well as a decreased consumption of flesh, other animal products , and the chemicals they contain. Truly, as one progresses towards a pure vegetarian diet, the cancer risk drops accordingly. Though developing cancer is common: it is not normal.

A Closer Look at the Alternatives

One study found that 95 to 99 percent of the chemicals in the Standard American Diet come from pork, beef, poultry, fish, dairy, and eggs.[180] Over ten times more pesticide residues can be found in beef, pork, poultry, and fish; and nine times more in dairy products, as compared to fruits.[181, 182] On top of this comes all the steroids, hormones and other drugs routinely injected into or fed to animals, as well as the high heavy metal levels within their tissues. All of these hazardous substances end up in the animal's flesh, eggs, and milk.

Mothers

A study published in *The New England Journal of Medicine*, found that the average pesticide level in the breast milk of vegetarian women was just one to two percent of the level found in non-vegetarian mothers.[183]

Organically Grown Foods

The Difference is in the Soil

Properly managed or cultivated "organic" gardens and farms have nutrient-rich soils due to beneficial worms, insects, and microorganisms, in addition to the natural compost provided by tree droppings and surrounding plants—a perfect, self-sustaining system (also see *Environmental Reasons for Fruit Consumption*). Healthy soil produces a healthy tree or plant, one with superior resistance to pests and disease. Conversely, beneficial creatures are non-existent in dead, poisoned soils, and the plants or trees produced in them are weak. Their fruits have poor ripening and pitiful keeping qualities. For example, supermarket tomatoes rot while they are still hard and pink.

Many of the seedless varieties of fruits (most or all of which are hybrids) require enormous amounts of pesticides during production (such as seedless grapes). Unfortunately, very few fruits (foods) have been un-tampered with through the centuries. The entire food supply is becoming increasingly corrupt, and one can only do their best from that which is available, remembering that raw fruits, nuts, seeds, vegetables, and other unprocessed plant foods are the safest to consume.

Nutrient-deficient soils *may* produce comparable nutrient value foods, but fewer in relation to the tree or plant; however, when a nutrient is lacking in the soil, it will be absent from the food. Therefore, when you cannot regulate the soil's nutrient balance (as in growing your own food) it makes sense to eat produce from a number of locales.

Growing Your Own
Why not cooperate with God and grow as much of your own food as possible? As compared to store-bought produce, homegrown fruits and vegetables are more flavorful, can be vine-ripened, freshly picked, and grown without pesticides; are higher in vitamins, minerals, and other nutrients; do not easily rot after harvest, are economical, and lessen dependence on others. Truly, gardening supplies most of the essentials for health: nutritious food, exercise, fresh air, sunshine, and spiritual and mental growth as one learns lessons from nature.

Suggestions for Obtaining Organically Grown Fruits
Visit farmer's markets and u-pick farms. Apples, pears, stone fruits, and other foods can be obtained at cheaper prices than those found in the supermarket. Do not be afraid to buy fruits with a few blemishes or wind scars. Just make sure that everything is mature and fresh—refer to the *Fruit Guide* for buying instructions.

Ask grocery stores in your area to stock organically grown produce. Many of the persimmons sold in supermarkets have been organically grown.

Organically grown, untreated dates and dried fruits can be obtained from a natural food distributor. Canadians will find it more feasible to start a buying club or co-op and to order through a Canadian-based bulk food distributor.

To verify whether the produce you are buying is organically grown check for proper certification (a sticker or stamp). California Certified Organic Farmers (CCOF) is a nonprofit trade association for organic farmers that requires growers to undergo a minimal three year transition period before qualifying for organic status. CCOF inspects member farms and packaging plants (if applicable) on a yearly basis. Other certification associations exist within North America; look them up if you have concerns about the produce that bears their certification.

What You Can Do To Greatly Reduce Your Intake Of Pesticides

1. Avoid flesh and other animal products.

2. Grow your own chemical-free produce.

3. Buy organically grown foods when they are competitively priced. Dried fruits should always be obtained from an organic source, and are affordable when purchased in bulk quantities.

4. Wash non-organically grown fruits and vegetables with warm water and produce soap (see below). Rinse or soak nuts and seeds.

5. Trim the skins off heavily waxed items such as apples and cucumbers.

6. Limit your intake of non-North American imports—avoiding sweet peppers, berries, tomatoes, stone fruits, and seedless grapes altogether.

7. Limit your intake of domestic peppers and berries (U.S. grown) and eschew seedless grapes (see *Grapes* in the *Fruit Guide*).

8. Rely heavily on thick-skinned fruits. Bananas, watermelons, mangos, oranges, avocados, and other thick-skinned fruits generally have the lowest pesticide levels in the flesh (pulp) itself.

9. Avoid commercially processed fruits and vegetables, including juices and canned produce (especially tomatoes).

10. Look for stickers that say "no pesticide residues detected."

Produce Soap

Produce soaps are recommended for use on all non-organically grown fruits and vegetables, particularly those whose edible portions have had direct exposure to pesticides.

Several companies in North America distribute non-toxic, animal product-free produce soaps, or all-purpose soaps that are suitable for use on fruits and vegetables. These may be purchased from health food stores or mail-order catalogs. Economy sizes are available.

Some Final Words

Do the best within your means, knowing that by eating a large percentage of raw, nutrient-rich fruits and vegetables and moderate amounts of nuts and seeds, that your body will possess the vitality necessary to combat poisonous agents. People who eat a preponderance of natural foods live longer, more abundant lives, often dying naturally of old age!

Obviously, one must use common sense and budget appropriately in order to properly feed a family. If organically grown fruits and vegetables cannot be obtained at reasonable prices in your area, and you are not able to grow your own at this time, be not dismayed, but do the best you can and focus on the One who said, "Therefore take no thought, saying, What shall we eat? or, What shall we drink? or, Wherewithal shall we be clothed? ...But seek ye first the kingdom of God, and his righteousness; and all these things shall be added unto you."

Genetic Engineering

Genetic engineering, an advanced form of biotechnology, involves the duplication or transferring of genes within plant and animal realms. Thousands of trials have been conducted on plants and animals. Currently, pigs are being "created" with human genes, tomatoes with salmon, flounder, bacteria, and virus genes; potatoes with chicken genes, crops with genes that enable them to be heavily treated with pesticides, and the list goes on.[184, 185, 186]

❑   *Human genes are actually being patented[187]—What must God think?*

For the most part, the general public has little knowledge regarding this disturbing technology, yet the products of it have already been forced into our food supply. Gene-altered foods are now being sold in supermarkets, and without requirements for labeling. Both American and Canadian citizens are eating genetically engineered "New Leaf" potatoes and "Flavor Savr" tomatoes, as well as corn, squash, soybean, and canola products. One major soup company intends to, or at this time is using the "Flavor Savr" tomato.

It has not stopped with genes: experiments with bacteria and viruses are also being conducted. This brings with it a whole list of additional risks that can only be hypothesized. When pesticides were first introduced, they too, were considered to be agriculture's problem-solver—ads were proudly stating "DDT is good for you."[188]

Milk, dairy products, and beef have been potentially hazardous to eat for decades, but since 1994, the stakes have been raised. Cows are being injected with recombinant bovine growth hormone (rBGH) in an attempt to increase milk production[189]—even though we already have storehouses of rotting dairy products. rBGH has been linked to breast and colon cancers, reproductive failures, and other diseases in cows,[190] and increases a persons chance of developing these same cancers.[191] *Children drink the most milk.* This contaminated milk is being consumed by American citizens, while Canadians are still trying to keep it off their shelves.

Irradiation

Irradiation is a process (classified as a food additive) that is used to extend the storage life of foods and to destroy microorganisms and pests. Sounds encouraging, but let us closely examine the facts.

Irradiation involves exposing foods to huge x-ray generators or to the radioactive materials Cobalt-60 (it's production generates nuclear waste) or Cesium-137 (a by-product of nuclear power and weapons). A single irradiation plant uses approximately 1000 times the Cesium-137 that was released by the bomb dropped on Hiroshima.[192] This opens up the possibility for some major accidents, not only at the plant, but during transport of the hazardous materials. Leaks can and do happen, like the one in Georgia in 1988 where milk, medical supplies, and contact lens solution had to be recalled.[193] One can only guess at the damage done to the workers, public, and environment.

When a food is subjected to radiation, its molecular structure becomes deranged: vitamins and enzymes are destroyed, fats become rancid, amino acids are altered, toxic chemicals and free radicals are formed, and new chemicals called URP's are developed.[194] Irradiated foods are still subject to aflatoxins, botulism, mutations, and recontamination, and still contain all the pesticides that were on the food before the treatment.[195]

❏   *Animals fed irradiated foods have high rates of infertility and still-births, kidney diseases, and tumors, and develop abnormal blood cells called polyploids which have been linked to leukemia. Sadly, with all this information available, irradiated foods were actually fed to malnourished children in India. The result: they developed the very same leukemia-linked cells that were formed in monkeys and other animals![196]*

Irradiation is not new, but rather has been promoted and used since the 1960's.[197] At this time, very few foods are being irradiated in North America. Spices and seasonings are always irradiated, and receive the highest doses by far—equivalent to 60 million chest x-rays! Spices also irritate and eventually destroy the natural sensitiveness of the stomach, make the blood feverish and impure, and weaken the moral and intellectual powers.[198, 199]

Poultry, fish, all other meats, potatoes, onions, and yams are the foods most likely to have been irradiated. Be watchful.

Protecting Yourself

At this time, a small flower symbol called the "radura," along with a statement indicating irradiation, is required on packaged (on the bag) and loosely sold produce (on the display sign). The law (U.S.) currently states that irradiated foods can be used as ingredients without being labeled as such. Therefore, the consumer would do well to avoid all processed foods, foods prepared outside the home, and whole foods identified as being irradiated. Imports also pose a threat.

The Radura

Chapter 5

More Environmental Reasons For Fruit Consumption

One's diet has an enormous impact on the environment, being in accordance with the laws that govern nature. Common sense tells us that a fruit-based diet will help to sustain this contaminated and damaged earth. We have been given the responsibility to tend the earth and keep it, so therefore we should work the land and live in such a manner as to maintain nature's equilibrium. Buying more fruits and nuts compels ranchers and farmers to make the transition to fruit and nut agriculture. In the United States, 64 percent of the cropland is used to grow feed for livestock, while only 2 percent is used to produce fruits and vegetables[200]—these figures should be reversed.

Orchards and other produce farms are highly efficient and non-depleting. Enormous quantities of food can be grown per acre of fruit or nuts. Orchards are superior because root systems hold the soil together, which means erosion is virtually non-existent. To complete this faultless system, droppings from the trees aid in fertilization, and the humus-rich soil retains moisture (less water needed). Can this perfect picture be any clearer? God created normal, natural food production in such a wonderful, flawless way as to let the earth replenish itself while providing man with a bountiful harvest. Of course, pesticides have no place in God's system because they poison the water, soil, air, and food.

Statistics

There is much more to this situation than meets the eye so let us investigate further. A comparison between tomatoes, apples, and one of North America's favorite foods—beef—will prove informative. An incredible 50,000 pounds (22 680 kg) of tomatoes or 20,000 pounds (9 072 kg) of apples can be produced per acre of land, as compared to beef where a mere 250 pounds (113.4 kg) of edible product may be obtained![201] In California, tomatoes require 23 gallons (87 liters) of water and apples 49 gallons (185 liters) to produce 1 pound (0.45 kg) of edible product, while beef demands a disgraceful 5,214 gallons (19 735 liters)![202]

To produce one day's worth of food for a meat-eater, it takes over 4,000 gallons (15 140 liters) of water, for a lacto-ovo vegetarian (eats dairy and eggs) 1,200 gallons (4 542 liters), and for a pure vegetarian just 300 gallons (1 135 liters).[203]

Approximately 90 percent of soy and 80 percent of the corn grown in the United States is fed to livestock.[204] To produce one pound of beef, it takes 16 pounds (7.3 kg) of soy and grain. Equivalents for other animal products are 16 pounds for chicken, 16 pounds for eggs, and 6 pounds (2.7 kg) for pork.[205] Over 22 million acres of prime soils have been destroyed beyond repair due to overgrazing, unsustainable farming practices, and deforestation.[206]

Other Major Impacts

Directly linked with the previous issues are soil erosion, carbon dioxide and methane emissions, water pollution from animal excrement and pesticides, and rain forest depletion.[207]

Chapter 6

Fruit Preservation

Drying

Drying is the oldest and most preferable method of food preservation. Advantages of dried fruits (and vegetables) include compact storage, lengthy storage times; high resistance to molds, bacteria, and pathogenic organisms; outstanding nutrient contents, super-sweet flavors, and they are even lightweight and travel-friendly. Another important factor is that organically grown dried fruits can be obtained at reasonable prices.

With drying, small quantities of nutrients are lost during the dehydration process, but the finished product (pound for pound) possesses three to six times the nutrients. Wherever possible, dried fruits should be a staple in the diet, particularly in the winter when more calories are needed. A dehydrator can be a beneficial investment for those who have their own fruit trees (or gardens), or who buy bulk quantities. Commercially sold dried fruits should be obtained from a natural food distributor who sells organically grown produce.

Home-drying allows one to enjoy a greater variety of dried fruits, and those who have children (of responsible age) can teach them some valuable skills. If you decide to dry some or all of your own fruit, avoid the use of sulphur and other chemical preservatives (see *Dried Fruits* in the *Fruit Guide* for an in depth discussion). Fruits that oxidize quickly may be pre-treated with lemon, lime, or orange juice. Buy a quality dehydrator and follow the instruction manual. Never attempt to dry fruits that are almost overripe.

Freezing

As compared to drying, freezing is a far less desirable method of food preservation because it causes a large percentage of vitamins to be destroyed; however, home-frozen fruits are preferable to those that have been commercially canned or frozen (these have been cooked and may contain additives and preservatives). All things considered, it is nice to home-freeze berries, persimmons and other short-season fruits (that withstand freezing well) for enjoyment throughout the year. Frozen foods should not constitute a large portion of one's diet.

Your freezer must be colder than -5°F (-21°C)—the colder, the better—to keep freezable fruits for the time periods listed in the *Fruit Guide*. Never use refined sugars or other harmful or unnatural preservatives, and to prevent fermentation, avoid overloading your freezer with too many freshly processed fruits. Use trays and racks to prevent bruising and the thawing of other foods, and place dated stickers on the freezer bags or plastic containers so that you can identify what needs to be used first. Leave expansion space in the bags or containers, and for convenience, freeze in ready-to-serve portions.

Chapter 7

Food Combining Principles

Food combining is the science pertaining to effective and efficient digestion of foodstuffs. Briefly stated, certain foods may be successfully eaten together because they have similar digestive requirements, thus allowing for thorough and efficient processing without the formation of poisonous waste products. Some types of foods are dissimilar yet still work well together due to corresponding digestive times, similar water contents, or even because one possesses a neutral character. With food combining, the length of time that various foods take to digest is the overriding factor to consider.

The object of food combining is twofold: to eat harmonious combinations of foods to prevent indigestion and the development of toxic by-products; and second, to allow for the maximal utilization of nutrients. Healthy blood equals a healthy body. Our study centers on fruits and nuts. The ideal situations are given unless stated otherwise. Keep in mind that while some people may thrive on a particular combination, others may have difficulty. All must use common sense and trial and error to determine the combinations that allow for the highest possible levels of mental and physical functioning.

Fruits with Other Foods
Fresh fruits are quickly processed by the body, passing through the stomach faster than all other types of food. Consequently, it makes sense to provide the

conditions that will allow fruits to make their journey without delay, thus preventing fermentation and the subsequent formation of poisonous alcohols. For the most part, when fruits are delayed in the stomach they ferment, while high-protein foods (animal products, legumes, or nuts) that are detained putrefy. Meals that contain foods other than fruits should be followed by at least five hours of abstinence before eating any type of food. Raw, enzyme-rich fruits are quickly digested, and when eaten in moderation and apart from other foods may be followed by a subsequent meal after four hours or less.

Desert the Dessert

Your stomach, brain, and entire body will be thankful if you avoid eating fruits after a non-fruit meal, especially one that contains milk (dairy), eggs, meats (this includes poultry and fish), and vegetables. The stomach should be empty before partaking of fruit. This can take from four to eight hours depending on the foods consumed at the previous meal, digestive vitality, and physical exertion. On the whole, animal products remain in the stomach the longest, followed by legumes, grains, starchy and non-starchy vegetables (some digest very quickly), nuts, seeds, dried fruits, fresh fruits, and melons. Taking melons or other fruits as a dessert results in fermentation and outright poisoning of the blood. This could actually cause death!

Fruits and Grains

Most people find well-cooked grains (toasted bread, oats, granola, millet, etc.) to combine harmoniously with fruits. Grains must be thoroughly cooked (toasted where applicable) and masticated (chewed), in order to convert starches into more-easily-digested disaccharides. This allows digestion to proceed more efficiently, thus preventing fermentation of the fruits. If you eat fruits and grains together, experiment to see which combinations work best. Fresh or dried fruits should be eaten raw whenever possible.

Fruits with Vegetables

For the most part, fruits and vegetables should never be combined. Tomatoes (if you class them as vegetables) would be an exception due to their consistency and rapid digestive time (about two hours). Also, those with good digestive powers have found dried fruits to combine well with plain, un-oiled lettuce since it is quickly digested and abundant in water. Oily fruits are also exempt from the fruit with vegetable rule.

Oily Fruits

Avocados, olives, and coconuts may be combined successfully with vegetables, starches, and most acid and sub-acid fruits. Those with strong digestive powers can eat them with sweet fruits. To prevent overeating and promote efficient digestion, oily fruits should not be eaten in large quantities, and for some, apart from other foods that are high in fat or protein (each other, legumes, nuts, seeds, or animal products). Nuts and seeds could also be placed in the oily fruits category, yet will be discussed later.

Sugars with Milk

Fruit (any type of sugar) taken with milk (any dairy product) represents one of the worst combinations. Dairy products form curds in the stomach and these prevent fruits (any foods) from being properly digested;[208] fermentation results, and this causes a plethora of poisonous wastes to enter the blood-stream. Realize that these toxins affect the brain and literally every cell in the body!

The extent that people violate this combination principle becomes evident when one considers some of the commonly eaten foods of today: ice creams, chocolate, milk shakes, yogurts, puddings, and sugar-coated cereals drenched in milk.

> ❑ *Taken alone, both milk and sugar increase blood fat levels, but when combined, this occurs to a much greater degree and remains so for up to ten hours![209] Milk and sugar combinations have also been shown to cause abnormally high levels of growth hormone.[210]*

Melons

Melons undergo rapid absorption and could cause distress if held up in the stomach by non-fruit foods, or even by sweet fruits such as bananas. Melons are best eaten alone as a meal in themselves. Freshly-squeezed juices and juicy fruits are the most acceptable items to combine with melons, but all must experiment for themselves.

Acid Fruits with Sweet Fruits

Is it okay to eat bananas and oranges together? If you do not experience distress, then eat with a good conscience. Secretions called buffers enable many people to handle acid and sweet fruits simultaneously.

Nuts and Seeds

Nuts and seeds may be combined with fruits, grains, and some types of vegeta-bles.[211] Most people will find nuts and seeds to combine well with tomatoes, citrus fruits, or berries. Others eat them with lettuce, cucumber, celery and like vegetables. Sub-acid fruits also combine reasonably well with nuts and seeds, but eating them with sweet fruits *could* prove troublesome for many. The rationale being that fat, protein, and sugar combinations appear to be ill-advised (see *Sugars with Milk*). Experiment to find out which fruits and vegetables combine effectively with nuts or seeds to allow for clear thinking and strength. Try one item at a time with *moderate* amounts of raw nuts or seeds. Most problems simply result from eating too many nuts.

Variety

The fewer varieties of fruits (or any foods) combined at a meal, the more efficient the digestion.

Chapter 8

Healthy Eating Tips

Tip #1 – Avoid Overeating!
Overeating suspends digestion and therefore causes foods to ferment or putrefy during the delay. Intoxication results, rather than nourishment.

Tip #2 – Slow Down!
Digestion begins in the mouth. Salivary enzymes only function effectively when foods have been thoroughly masticated. At least twenty-five minutes should pass before a meal has been completed.

Tip #3 – Limiting the Number of Meals
Eat just two or three meals per day and allow enough time between meals so that the stomach can empty its contents before being summoned into action again.

Tip #4 – Eat a Good Breakfast
Plan your eating schedule so that you will be ready for a good breakfast in the morning. Breakfast and midday meals should be the largest of the day, while supper, if taken at all, should be light and even less complicated. Obviously, one must use common sense and plan meals according to the type of labor (mental, light work, or heavy physical) as well as the weather conditions. If

one must do mental labor in the morning and physical labor in the afternoon, then perhaps the midday meal could be the largest?

Tip #5 – Frequency and Timing

Eating at regular times allows the digestive organs to prepare secretions and to be ready for duty. Avoid eating within four hours before bedtime—six hours if you have chosen to make your final meal heavy. The functioning of the digestive system is hampered during the night, and laying in a horizontal position prevents efficient digestion. Gravitational forces cause food to remain in the upper portion of the stomach, sometimes forcing it back into the esophagus—heartburn and acid throat result.

Eating immediately before strenuous exercise or work is contraindicated because the blood will be driven from the digestive organs to the muscles. The same principle applies to eating before mental exertion such as an exam (the blood being driven to the brain). Mild physical exertion such as casual walking or light manual work will prove to be an aid to digestion.

Tip #6 – Limiting the Numbers of Foods

Limiting the varieties of foods at a meal allows for efficient digestion and prevents overeating.

Tip #7 – Eschew All Foods Between Meals

Even a bite of something triggers the draining of digestive secretions. Snacking also interferes with the processing of the previous meal.

Tip #8 – Only Eat When Truly Hungry

Hunger is a mouth, throat, and overall body sensation and not a grumbling stomach. Our stomachs have not been designed to work 24 hours a day, and therefore they need time to recuperate. A properly designed eating and living schedule will have you coming to the table hungry.

Hunger is generally absent during illness, an obvious sign to abstain from food and to let the body use all the available energy for restoration, rather than in the processing of foodstuffs. A day or more of fasting, taking only distilled water, will accelerate the healing process. Of course, one should strive to live in a manner that eliminates sickness altogether.

Tip #9 – Avoid Eating When Emotionally Upset

Emotional upsets prevent normal functioning of the digestive apparatus.

Tip #10 – When Exhausted, Skip the Next Meal

The body requires more energy for digestion than almost any other function, so do not force it into action when you are tired. Passing up an evening meal (or snack) encourages sound sleep and ensures hunger upon arising.

Tip #11 – Water

Drinking water fifteen minutes or more before a meal clears out the residues from the previous meal and helps to curb the appetite. If one's meal (or overall diet) consists largely of fruit, especially melons, then extra water may not even be required (unless the weather is extremely hot). Drinking fluids with a meal hinders enzymatic activity.

Tip #12 – Avoiding Hazards

Throw out foods that have uncharacteristic flavors or odors, and those with visible signs of mold. Eliminate dietary abominations such as alcohol, caffeine (coffee, tea, sodas, chocolate, etc.), condiments, spices, animal flesh, refined grains, fermented foods, highly saturated fats, products that contain vinegar, and junk foods (candy, donuts, etc.).

Immediately prior to consumption or preparation, wash pesticides and dirt from all types of produce (see *What You Can Do To Greatly Reduce Your Intake Of Pesticides*).

Kitchen Safety — Food Contamination

All kinds of flesh foods represent the greatest contamination hazard in the kitchen—by far. Salmonella is the most common threat but there are many others, most of which are potentially lethal (see *Factory Farmed Animals and Disease*). Eggs and dairy products are responsible for most of the remaining contamination hazards associated with foods. Once again, salmonella is the greatest danger (see *Ice Cream* in the Recipe section). Obviously, eliminating all flesh foods would drastically reduce ones risk of disease due to contamination (as well as cancer, heart disease, etc.), and abstaining from animal products altogether would be the easy way to avoid practically every life-threatening food-related disease that plagues society (if one prepares their own food in a clean kitchen).

However, those who choose to eat flesh, eggs, or dairy products can take some precautions to minimize the risk for themselves, those who they prepare food for, and all others who must use the same kitchen. Detailed information regarding the numerous safety precautions in buying, storing, thawing, cooking, serving, and post cleanup of animal products can be obtained from the government or a library.

Bacteria such as salmonella cannot be killed by hot water.[212] At all times when handling flesh and eggs, a thorough cleanup must be performed. To be brief, all cutlery, cutting boards, plates and dishes, counters, sinks, and hands that come in contact with raw flesh or eggs, or with any of the items that do, should be sterilized with a chlorine bleach solution (see directions on bottle. About 5 ml bleach to 1L of water[213]). As stated in the section on water, chlorine is a carcinogen. Whether one takes it in through water or the lungs makes no difference. So, one threat (contamination) is exchanged for another; however, bleaching eliminates the immediate hazard, especially for those who can evacuate the premises. Bleaching should be done immediately after all the potentially hazardous foods have been handled, and before raw foods are prepared. Windows should be wide open for thorough oxygen exchange, and children and all others should be given the opportunity to leave the residence. To say the least, precious time is lost and the expense to the health of those involved is inestimable.

Other potential food contaminants include botulism toxin (home and commercially-canned foods, and honey) and aflatoxins (see *Peanuts*). Thankfully, most living in North America can obtain (or grow) a wide variety of fresh produce year-round, and therefore have no need to rely on canned foods, and to the benefit of superior nutrition and safety (see *Canned Fruits* for more). If canned foods are used, look for signs of spoilage when you open the can: unpleasant odors, spurting, or foaming. Do not even taste the food, but wrap the can in plastic bags, refrigerate, and contact health authorities.

Cooked grains, legumes, and vegetables, and raw prepared produce can be potentially harmful when stored incorrectly.

Part 2

The Practical Fruit Guide

Introduction

In the following pages you will learn everything needed to acquire the safest and most flavorful fruits. The guide is teeming with little-known shopping, storing, preparation, and health tips, as well as interesting facts. The illustrations add beauty and clarify each fruit's description.

Buying suggestions are listed for every fruit, but the reader is encouraged to grow as much of their own produce as possible. Home-grown produce is more flavorful, higher in vitamins, minerals, and all other nutrients (when the soil is properly managed); can be vine-ripened, freshly picked, and grown without pesticides, does not easily rot after harvest, is economical, and prevents dependence on others. Additional benefits include exercise, fresh air, sunshine, and lessons from nature. The miraculous creative powers that govern nature never fail to astonish and teach the gardener. Everyone can grow something, even in planters, buckets, or jars. Teaching your children how to grow their own food and allowing them to learn from nature is of utmost importance. Self-sufficiency in food production may not be realistic, and is unwise for those living in climates where few fruits can be grown, but one should always strive to grow something. Nevertheless, to learn how to make quick, knowledgeable decisions at the market, frequently refer to this guide or even take it to the market until you are familiar with every fruit.

Each fruit described bears one of the following classifications: sweet, sub-acid, acid, melon, protein, starch, or neutral. These classifications have been provided for those who use food combining principles (see *Food Combining*), and denote the predigested characters, not the true residue left upon metabolism: an orange is classed *acid* but leaves an alkaline ash (for an in depth discussion, refer to *Acid-Base Balance*, and *Raw vs. Cooked* in Part 1).

Exotic fruits have been included for those who can grow or obtain them at reasonable prices (whether home or away). The symbols used in the *Practical Fruit* and *Recipe Guides* can be quickly accessed from the following legend.

🖉	Noteworthy tips and suggestions.
☠	Chemicals and other hazards.
💣	Definite avoidances.
🗁	Health information.
✍	Interesting facts.

Tips At A Glance

The following tips just touch on those outlined throughout the remainder of the book. Many more will be revealed as you explore each fruit.

Tip #1 – Peak Season Fruits
For superior quality and lower prices, select fruits during peak and semi-peak seasons. Don't think twice about avoiding that imported melon or peaches in the winter.

Tip #2 – High Quality
Purchase high quality fruits. Shun immature, overripe, or damaged produce.

Tip #3 – Color and Weight
Always select characteristically colored, heavy fruits because this indicates maturity, high juice content, and freshness.

Tip #4 – Using Your Senses
When shopping, use all of your senses: sight for outer appearance, touch for gentle squeezing (such as melons) and gauging weight, smell to determine ripeness or possible fermentation, and hearing to listen for sloshy, overripe melons.

Tip #5 – Hybrids
The author avoids all "new fruits"—those that have been developed by man through crossing two different fruits together. For example, a tangerine would be purchased, but not a tangelo (a tangerine-pummelo cross). Seedless varieties (watermelons, grapes, etc.) are "weak" (see *Grapes*), and whenever possible, should be avoided in favor of non-hybrid seeded varieties. For those who wish to bypass crossed fruits, indications have been added throughout the *Fruit Guide* wherever a definite identification has been made. Know that the author is unaware of every hybrid. Very few fruits (foods) have been un-tampered with through the centuries, and much research would be required to locate those that are true to their original species. One must keep in mind that fruits are superior to the hazardous alternatives.

Tip #6 – Wise Shopping
Buy bulk quantities for better prices. It is rarely a mistake to buy cases, flats, and boxes of fruit because extra can always be dried or frozen. Split large orders with family or friends. Organically grown and other more expensive fruits such as mangos suddenly become affordable when bought in greater quantities.

Tip #7 – Wise Shopping

To prevent unnecessary bruising and damage, take boxes to the market for loading fruits (even the melons).

Tip #8 – Wise Shopping

Shop around. Buy from grocery stores, wholesalers, co-ops (start your own), and farms. Develop friendships with suppliers and growers in your area. Look for specials. Spend a few minutes each week checking the produce ads. Ninety-five percent of the advertised fruit will be "in-season," and therefore of excellent quality.

Tip #9 – Hazards

To prevent possible contamination (salmonella etc.), place all fresh produce items in plastic bags before running them over the grocery check-out belt—fruits and most vegetables are (or should be) eaten raw, and salmonella needs to be killed with bleach, a carcinogen that should never be used to clean food. Use produce soap and warm water to clean fruits and vegetables.

Shun genetically engineered and irradiated fruits (foods).

To avoid temptation while shopping, gather the fruits, vegetables, and other natural foods that are essential—and straightway leave the store.

Tip #10 – Ripening

Ripen fruits at room temperature. Place them in paper bags to accelerate the ripening process, and add bananas for even quicker results.

Tip #11 – Storage

To prevent spoilage (molds or fermentation), know what fruits you have, how to store them, and how long they will keep. In unforeseen circumstances you can always dry or freeze excess.

Do not store unripe fruits in the refrigerator—those fruits that keep well in cold storage (pears, etc.) may be kept cold up to a point.

To prevent tearing of the peel and bruising, remove stickers from persimmons, tomatoes, pears, and stone fruits before they become ripe.

Tip #12 – Cutting Frozen Fruit

Exercise extreme caution when cutting frozen fruit and use a warm knife to prevent difficulties.

Thanks to the Australian Rare Fruit Counsel for helping to fill in some of the gaps on several of the exotic fruits.

Fruits Listed in Order of Appearance

Abiu
Acerola
Akee
Apple
Apricot
Asian Pear
Atemoya
Avocado
Babaco
Bananas and Plantains
Berries
    Blackberry
    Boysenberry
    Loganberry
    Blueberry
    Cranberry
    Currant
    Gooseberry
    Huckleberry
    Jaboticaba
    Limeberry
    Mulberry
    Raspberry
    Strawberry
Black Sapote
Breadfruit
Cacao
Cactus Fruit
Caimito
Canistel
Carissa Plum
Carob
Ceriman

Cherimoya
Cherry
Citrus
    Citron
    Grapefruit
    Kumquat
    Lemon
    Lime
    Oranges
    Temple Orange
    Tangerines
    Tangelos
    Mandarins
    Pummelo
    Ugli
Coconut
Date
Durian
Feijoa
Fig
Grapes
Guava
Inga
Jakfruit
Kiwano
Kiwi
Litchi or Lychee
Longan
Loquat
Mabolo
Mamey
Mammea
Mango

Fruits Listed in Order of Appearance

Mangosteen
Melons
   Honeydew
   Sharlyne
   Crenshaw
   Cantaloupe
   Nutmeg
   Casaba
   Persian
   Juan Canary
   Watermelon
Mombin
Nectarine
Olive
Papaya
Passion Fruit
Paw Paw
Peach
Pears
Persimmon
Physalis
Pineapple
Pitanga
Pitomba
Plum
Pomegranate
Quince
Rambutan
Ramontchi
Sapodilla
Soursop
Star Fruit

Sugar Apple
Tamarind
Tamarillo
Vanilla
Wampee
Water Apple
White Sapote
Dried Fruits
   Raisins, all others
Nuts and Seeds
   Almonds
   Brazil
   Cashew
   Chestnut
   Filberts
   Macadamia
   Peanut
   Pecan
   Pine Nut
   Pistachio
   Walnut
   Pumpkin Seeds
   Sesame Seeds
   Sunflower Seeds
Vegetable-fruits
   Cucumber
   Eggplant
   Sweet Pepper
   Summer Squash
   Tomato

The Practical Fruit Guide

Abiu (Pouteria caimito)

Indigenous to the Amazon River Basin, the abiu is an apple-sized, yellow fruit whose exterior resembles that of a grapefruit. Severing the thick peel reveals pale yellow, jelly-like, glistening flesh. One to four large seeds are situated near the center. The flavor and texture can be likened to muskmelon and persimmon blended together.
Buying: Select fully-colored, softening fruits because immature ones contain latex near the skin.
Season: Summer.
Storing: Ripe abiu may be refrigerated for several days.
Serving: Halve and eat with a spoon, quarter and use a fork, or simply eat out of hand.
Class: Sweet

Acerola (Malpighia glabra)
Common Names: Barbados, Puerto Rican, or West Indian cherry

The acerola is a bright red, tart berry about half the size of a cherry. Native growing areas include Tropical America and the West Indies.
Season: Spring through fall.
Nutrients: The highest source of vitamin C known to man *—twenty-six times that of the orange!*
Class: Acid

Akee (Blighia sapida)
Common Name: Vegetable brain

The akee is an exotic tree-grown fruit native to Africa. It has pale yellow or reddish skin and ripens while hanging on the tree, as evidenced by separation at its seams, which reveals three large brown seeds and oily yellow flesh. The akee's skin, seeds, and even the flesh (at times) are poisonous! The flesh can only be eaten when firm.

Buying: *Avoid akee unless certain of its stage of ripeness. Unripe and overripe fruits could cause death!* Africa, Jamaica, and other tropical regions grow akee.

Class: Sub-acid

Apple (Malis pumila)

Apples are some of the most popular fruits due to their availability, long-lasting properties, and reasonable prices. Some 7000 to 9000 varieties exist, so we can only scratch the surface here.

These ancient fruits made their way from China to England through Roman conquest. Explorers brought apples to the "new world," and in 1629, pilgrims planted seeds at Massachusetts Bay.[1]

Apples are closely related to pears, peaches, plums, nectarines, and cherries. The trees lie dormant during the winter, showing life in the spring with leaf and flower buds. Bees pollinate the flowers.

⬾ Apples develop size and color during the summer months, but the true ripening occurs in the fall. Sweetness manifests during the last couple of weeks before harvesting when the tree discontinues the fruit's food supply.[2] Growers must wait for full sugaring to occur before harvesting the fruits.

Buying: Select firm, un-bruised apples with full coloring as indicated by the variety—not shiny wax. Apples should smell like apples! Those that yield to pressure have mealy flesh. For the best flavor and keeping qualities, pick medium-sized fruits unless the variety indicates otherwise (see varieties). Handle gently to prevent bruising and unnecessary waste.

Storing: Apples should be crisp and juicy but these qualities are soon lost through improper storage. They must be kept in a cold, humid atmosphere, either in the refrigerator or a cold storage room. Apples destined for the refrigerator should be placed in plastic bags to retard breakdown and prevent the absorption of undesirable odors. Those kept in a cold storage room do well in covered containers—be sure to cull them frequently because one or two bad apples can ruin the whole lot.

Commercial apples are monitored under controlled atmosphere conditions. Storage life is lengthened by slowing the respiration rate through reduced temperature and oxygen deprivation—similar to home storage but an exact science.

☠ Almost all supermarket apples are heavily coated in wax (For the hazards of waxes, see *Obtaining Safe Food* in Part 1). Apples should be eaten with the skins as was intended, because the highest concentrations of vitamins and minerals lie near the skins; however, eating the skins is contraindicated whenever waxes have been applied. Soaking apples in warm water will quickly reveal whether waxes have been used. Paring waxed apples substantially lowers one's intake of pesticides. Organically grown apples can be obtained at cheaper or comparable prices through direct contact with farmers. Better yet, plant some apple trees. Do the best within your means, remembering that non-organically grown produce is superior to animal products and refined foods.

Nutrients: A good source for potassium.

Class: Sub-acid

❑   *The following varieties are listed in alphabetical order according to the author's initial research.*

Braeburn
Super crisp and crunchy with a delectable sweet taste. Medium to extra-large with red and pale-green skin. Excellent storage qualities. Originated in New Zealand by crossing a Lady Hamilton and a Granny Smith.

Cortland
Similar to the McIntosh in appearance, but less flavorful—red blush with white tangy-sweet flesh. Commercially grown in Nova Scotia.

Elstar
A juicy, tangy-sweet apple with a fruity aroma and creamy texture. Yellowish-green and almost fully flushed with red or orange. Available for six months post harvest but superior during the first month.

Empire
A bright red, deliciously sweet, crisp fruit. Developed in New York as a cross between a McIntosh and a Red Delicious. The Empire does not have the juiciness of a McIntosh, but its crispness may be preferred. For best flavor, buy during the fall.

Fuji
A fine apple with crisp, sweet flesh. Developed by crossing a Ralls Janet with a Delicious. Select heavily blushed fruits for characteristic flavoring. Excellent keeping qualities.

Gala
An attractive, medium-sized apple with crisp, sweet, juicy flesh. Yellow and heavily flushed in red. New Zealand Galas are outstanding for flavor.

Golden Delicious
A superb fruit with crisp, juicy, uniquely sweet flesh. Excellent keeping qualities allow for year-round consumption, but for superior flavor, buy during the first four months after harvest. Originated in West Virginia. Often reasonably priced.

Granny Smith
This Australian native is extremely firm, crisp, and juicy, and possesses an unmistakable tart bite. Warrants a year-round classification because it stores well and is grown on both sides of the world.

Gravenstein
An irregularly shaped apple with green base coloring and light to heavy red blush. The flesh is semi-smooth and tangy-sweet, similar to a Macintosh. Commercially grown in Nova Scotia.

Grimes golden
A large, golden to yellow apple. Tangy-sweet.

Jonagold
A large, juicy, mildly sweet fruit. Greenish-yellow skin with red blush. Developed by crossing a Golden Delicious and a Jonathan. Jonagolds store poorly, bruising easily and becoming mushy.

Jonathan
A small, crisp, tangy apple with origins in New York. Drawbacks include easy bruising and brief storage.

Macintosh
An Ontario native whose fine flavor, creamy texture, and reasonable prices has earned it a place among the top five apples produced in North America. Macintosh apples bruise very easily so handle them appropriately. Coloring: red blush on green skins.

Newton
Firm and crisp with a sterling tart flavor. The perfect choice for those who like crunch. Yellowish-green skins. Best from September to January.

Northern Spy
A large fruit with firm, tangy flesh. Yellowish-green and flushed with red. Buy during the first two months after harvest.

Red Delicious
The most widely grown variety in North America due to its appearance and keeping qualities. The streaked or solid red skins look beautiful, but sadly, the tart-sweet flesh tends to be flavorless, dry, and woody.

Spartan
A crisp, sweet, succulent fruit with bright white flesh and a very small core. High quality for up to four months post harvest. Inexpensive at certain times of the season.

Stayman
A tart, juicy, reddish-purple fruit with excellent storage qualities. Daughter of the Winesap. Buy until January.

Winesap
A crisp, juicy, thick-skinned fruit with reddish-purple skin and tart, juicy flesh. Keeps very well.

Others
Rome Beauty, York Imperial, Rhode Island Greening, and Crab apples.

❏ *Places of origin provided by the International Apple Institute and B.C. Tree Fruits.*

Apricot *(Prunus armeniaca)*

The apricot is an ancient species thought to be cultivated in China over 3000 years ago. The fruits are small, spherical or oval, and fuzzy, with beautiful hues of orange, gold, or pink. When ripe, their deep orange flesh is soft and mildly sweet. Apricots are freestone, meaning that the stone does not cling to the flesh.

Buying: Apricots bruise easily, so choose those free from soft spots. To ensure complete development: select plump specimens with full, deep coloring. Check around the stem for undesirable tinges of green. Look for apricots with the stems intact, and examine all others for signs of interior decay. Immature, poorly-colored fruits and "flesh-rot" are major problems with out-of-season imports —*avoid them altogether!* Apply the above guidelines to all stone fruits.

The widely cultivated *Perfection* is a fine, golden to deep orange apricot with outstanding flavor. There are several other excellent varieties available.
Season: June through August.
Storing: Ripe apricots yield easily to gentle pressure. At this point, place them on a plate or suitable flat surface and refrigerate for up to one week.
Drying: Dry in halves or quarters. A delicious, super-concentrated source of carotene.
Freezing: Wash gently, halve, remove the stones, and place into freezer bags or plastic containers. Use within six months.
Nutrients: An outstanding source for beta carotene—the non-toxic, natural precursor of vitamin A that is abundant in all orange and yellow fruits. Significant amounts of vitamin C, folic acid, niacin, silicon, and potassium.
Class: Sub-acid

Asian Pear (Pyrus pyrifolia)

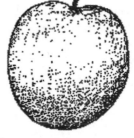

As the name implies, Asian pears are native to Japan and China. Surprisingly, they share more characteristics with apples than pears, being crisp and firm when ripe and almost spherical in shape. The flavor is a mix between the two, leaning more towards a pear. Asian pears have golden or yellow skins with a texture similar to the Bosc pear.

✎ European pears are more flavorful and less expensive.
Buying: Select firm, fully-colored fruits.
Storing: Keep in the crisper for up to three weeks.
Season: November through April.
Class: Sub-acid

Atemoya (Annona squamosa x Annona cherimola)

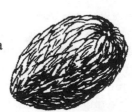

The atemoya is a member of the *annona* family. It is a cross between a sugar apple and a cherimoya, and therefore, being a hybrid, will not be recommended to the reader. The original fruits should be sought after.
Class: Sweet

Avocado *(Persea americana, P. gratissima)*
Common Name: Alligator pear

Avocados are native to Central America, and have steadily gained popularity due to their rich buttery flavors. There are well over 100 varieties having different shapes, sizes, flesh and skin colors, as well as tastes. Avocados may be pear-shaped, round, oval, or resemble a crookneck squash. Miniatures weigh just a couple of ounces (57 g), while mammoth fruits often exceed five pounds (2.3 kg). The bumpy or smooth skins exhibit varying shades of green, and the creamy flesh may be exceptionally flavored or bland. A large, tightly-enclosed or loosely-held seed is responsible for the bulbous appearance.

Buying: *Always purchase fully green unripe avocados!* Avocados bruise easily, and when roughly handled, spoilage is soon to follow.

🌢 Avoid unripe avocados that have been kept cold (blackening fruits that are still very firm) because they will never develop full potential.

A Better Choice: Avocados have *very* low pesticide residues.

Storing: Avocados must be ripe prior to refrigeration. At this point they keep for up to five days (depending upon the variety). Ripen at room temperature until they yield to *very gentle* pressure. For quicker results: place avocados in a paper bag with some bananas.

Serving: Avocados are great right from the shell, as guacamole, in dressings and salsas (see *Recipes*), or in place of butter, mayonnaise, margarine, and any other spread that is high in saturated fat. Once you start using avocados in these ways, you will never go back to the less flavorful, health corrupting alternatives.

✐ To prevent bruising: place ripe avocados small bowls before refrigerating.

Nutrients: An excellent source for thiamine, riboflavin, niacin, pantothenic acid, pyridoxine, potassium, chlorine, and sulphur. Significant amounts of carotene, vitamin C, silicon, and magnesium.

🗁 Avocados contain a high percentage of monounsaturated fat, which has been shown to discourage high cholesterol levels when eaten in moderation.

Class: Neutral, protein-fat

❑ Avocados listed according to richness of flavor.

Haas
The Haas is the most popular variety of avocado due to its superlative flavor and rich, buttery consistency. These characteristics are the result of a high fat

content—cholesterol free. The pear-shaped fruits have thick, heavily pebbled, dark green skins, which generally turn black upon ripening. The Haas possesses excellent storage qualities, and once ripe, may be refrigerated for up to five days. A combination of Californian and Mexican harvests allows for availability eleven months of the year. Peaks from April to December.

Sharwill

A large, semi-bumpy, pear-shaped fruit with excellent flavor. Available during the late summer and early fall. The Sharwill is generally the most expensive avocado.

Reed

A rounded avocado with an extra large seed. The flesh is creamy and full-flavored. Available during the fall.

Florida Avocados

Florida avocados have smooth, bright green skins during the summer, and rough skins in the winter. A large number of varieties exist as evidenced by the assortment of shapes and sizes. Some are over a foot in length and shaped like crookneck squashes. The diverse flavors of Florida avocados are very good for the most part, with some being excellent, although none can compare to the Haas. Florida avocados are less flavorful because they contain a greater percentage of water and a lower quantity of fat. Available July through March.

Fuerte

A pear-shaped avocado with smooth green skin and a fine, although light, flavor. Look for Fuertes from October through March.

Zutano

The Zutano is a smooth, pear-shaped avocado with thin skin. Its flavor is mild due to the high water content of the flesh. Fall and winter availability.

Bacon

A smooth, pear-shaped avocado with thin skin. Possesses a light flavor due to the higher water content of its flesh. Available during the fall and winter. Does not store well.

Babaco *(Carica babaco, C. pentagona)*

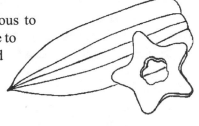

The babaco is a peculiar fruit indigenous to
Ecuador. It bears a striking resemblance to
the star fruit (carambola) as evidenced
by its fluted form. Individuality
resides in expanded dimensions, a
hollowed center, rounded edges, and
preferable flavor. Lengths of 10 inches
(25 cm) are common. Fully ripe
babacos possess bright yellow or golden skins and juicy-sweet yellow flesh.
Buying: Select firm fruits with at least 50 percent color. New Zealand
produces a commercial crop.
Storing: When ripe, wrap in a towel (prevents chilling) and place in the
crisper for up to two days.
Serving: Slice horizontally to create star-shaped rounds.
Drying: Dry as "stars."
Nutrients: An excellent source for vitamin C.
Class: Sub-acid

Bananas and Plantains

(Musa acuminata, M. paradisiaca)

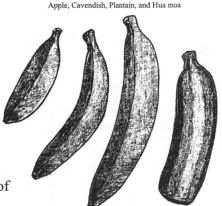

Apple, Cavendish, Plantain, and Hua moa

The banana is the world's most
popular fruit due to its sweet flavor,
availability, convenience, and
inexpensiveness. It is not surprising that such a perfect food also
happens to be one of the oldest,
dating back at least 500 years before
the birth of Jesus.[3] Perhaps bananas
were growing in Eden? Arabs spoke of
the plant as the "tree of paradise."[4]

A Spanish missionary is credited with bring-
ing the banana west to Santo Domingo via
the Canary Islands.[5] Today, all tropical countries grow bananas with North
American supplies coming from Central and South America. Hawaii and
Florida produce small crops.

Surprisingly, the banana is not a tree but a giant herbaceous plant having
one growing point (a monocot).[6] The stem is a shallow-rooted pseudobulb
whose leaves and fruit emerge from the center and up through the top. The

pseudobulb produces auxiliary buds that develop into suckers which eventually grow to produce their own fruit.[7] A properly tended banana planting possesses a full-sized, fruit-bearing plant, one ¾ grown, another ¼ mature, and a sucker just breaking the soil. This "family" is called a mat. It takes from 9 to 14 months for a plant to produce fruit.[8] As bananas hang from the plant they are called *heads* or *bunches*. Bunches are cut into *hands* that have eight or more bananas, or *clusters* with three to seven *fingers*.

Bananas give off ethylene gas as they ripen, which stimulates enzymatic activity within, causing starches to be converted into easily digestible sugars. The pulp becomes soft and the skin color gradually transforms from green to yellow. A totally green banana contains about 20 percent starch and less than 2 percent sugar, while a brown-speckled, ripe fruit has reversed percentages.[9] The conversion of starch to sugars occurs throughout the ripening process, but the greatest changes take place as the color becomes fully yellow and starts to speckle.

Virtually all the bananas in our supermarkets have been artificially treated with ethylene gas to rush the ripening process. Thankfully, bananas have been created with thick peels.

✐ Use the small amounts of ethylene naturally given off by bananas to stimulate the ripening of other fruits or the bananas themselves. Simply place the desired number of bananas into a paper bag, alone, or with any other fruits. To prevent loss from bruising, separate the bunches.

If you purchase large quantities of bananas and need to stagger the ripening times, ripen them at different temperatures: keep some in the basement (anywhere slightly cooler), others on the countertop, and if needed, ripe ones in the refrigerator.

A Better Choice: Bananas have very low pesticide residues, and therefore should be a staple in everyone's diet.

Selecting/Storing: Purchase greater quantities of bananas during the winter when prices are lower and fewer varieties of peak-season domestic fruits are available.

Choosing solid green fruits reduces the chance of bruising. Bananas bruise much easier than people realize and must be handled accordingly. Bruising, the resulting soft spots, and fermentation often occur without visible damage to the peel. If you prefer to buy a yellowing hand: check for discoloration and softening. Take boxes into the supermarket for loading bananas and other fruits, being sure that they are handled gently. Grocery carts have not been designed with fruits and vegetables in mind.

Buying near-ripe bananas allows one to more accurately determine whether proper temperatures were provided during transport and storage. Avoid those having a dull, grayish complexion (indicating subjection to cold temperatures) because these may not develop to perfection (they will ripen but the flavor may not be quite as sweet). It is difficult to judge the degree of ripeness with chilled fruits. Speckles will only develop sparingly and the ends could remain green. Eat these when they yield to gentle pressure.

Bananas subjected to high temperatures have soft pulp and poor peel integrity. The peels show splits and the stems are weak, partially or entirely breaking away.

🖉 Select large, plump fruits (for the particular variety) as these have greater maturity and therefore possess superior flavor and nutrient content. They are also a better value because the thickness of the peel is the same for all sizes.

Bananas often considered as "overripes" (well-speckled) are at their peak—perfect for fresh eating and freezing. Buy overripes if they are inexpensive and appear to be in good condition. Excess can be refrigerated, dried, frozen, or shared.

🖉 Refrigerate fully ripe (speckled) bananas for up to five days when you need to extend the storage life. The peels become discolored but the fruit remains undamaged—this applies to unbruised bananas that have been placed gently on a plate or suitable flat surface.

📁 Bananas are one of the first non-breast foods given to babies due to their consistency, ease of digestion, sweetness, non-allergenic properties, and high nutrient content. *Surprisingly, the protein content of bananas is nearly equivalent to that of mother's milk!*

Serving: See the recipe section to discover the versatility of the banana. Of course, it cannot be more satisfying than to eat bananas right from the peel as they have been provided in nature.

〰 Have you ever had difficulty in peeling a banana? We can learn from monkeys: these experts peel them from the non-stem end and never have a problem.

Drying: Dried bananas are a super-sweet treat. Dry them whole, in strips, or as chewy or crunchy chips. Rehydrate whole ones or strips until they are soft on the outside and chewy in the center. Use distilled water so that the super-sweet *banana juice* will be fit to drink.

Freezing: Bananas freeze extremely well and can be used to make ice cream and shakes (see *Recipes*). When fully ripe, peel and place them (single-layer-high) into resealable freezer bags, removing the excess air. Freeze flat. You can also freeze unpeeled bananas—for easy removal of the peel, briefly soak them in a bowl of warm water.

Nutrients: An excellent source for potassium and vitamin B_6. Significant amounts of vitamin C.

Class: Sweet

Apple (Manzano)
Short, plump, and often referred to as a "finger" banana. As the name indicates, it has a mildly sweet, banana-apple flavor. Look for Apple bananas in natural food stores, specialty markets, and when visiting tropical countries.

Brazilian
A small, deliciously sweet finger banana.

Cavendish
The basic store-bought fruit. Outstanding sweet flavor.

Gros Michelle
The Gros Michelle used to be the principle variety found in supermarkets, but is only produced on a small scale today due to its susceptibility to fungus.

Ice Cream (Blue Java)
A beautiful fruit with powdery, turquoise-green skin. Fine, sweet flavor.

Lacatan
Comparable to the Cavendish in appearance and taste.

Macaboo (Red)
Short, medium to large, thick fruits with dark red skin. The dense pulp is smooth and slightly darker than the standard Cavendish. Unsurpassed flavor! Known by many names including Jamaican Red, Cuban Red, Morado, Indio, and Hawaiian Red.[10]

Macaboo (Green)
A Red Macaboo with green skin.

Musa Velutina
This head of fruit appears to be from another world because it grows straight up from the top of the plant and consists of tiny, bright pink, furry bananas. The flavor is said to be sweet, although the pulp contains a number of rock-hard seeds.[11]

Mysore
A small, chubby, slightly curved fruit with a sweet, rich flavor.

Orinoco (Horse)
An unmistakably ridged and thick banana with little or no curvature and sharply tapered ends. Sweet, mild acid flavor. A fully ripe, peeled "Horse" banana bends over when held upright from one end.

Praying Hands
A perfect name for an incredible head of fruit whose fingers are fused together to form the appearance of "praying hands." Undoubtedly, the work of a masterful Designer! The fused fingers are easily pulled from the hands as they ripen. Superlative, sweet flavor.

Thousand Finger
Another wondrous work of creation. The head is a breathtaking sight to behold, growing to a remarkable length of 9 feet (3 m) and possessing over 1000 miniature bananas! Peeled fruits are just $1\frac{1}{2}$ inches (2-3 cm) long. Sweet to sub-acid flavor.

Plantains

Giant & Dwarf Plantains
Plantains are longer and thicker than bananas, and have greater firmness and dense creamy pulp. Their uniquely rich, sweet flavor is very satisfying. Plantains are commonly, but mistakenly, thought to be cooking bananas. They can and should be eaten raw in order to obtain all of the vital enzymes and other nutrients that are destroyed or altered by cooking. Cooked plantains taste bland, so to impart flavor, undesirable ingredients are usually added such as fat, sugar, eggs, milk, butter, and spices.

The secret to eating raw plantains is *patience*. The starches need time to be completely converted into sugars. This takes much longer than with bananas because plantains have lower moisture contents. The Plantain has approximately 65 percent water, while the banana contains about 75 percent. Ripe plantains yield to pressure and have partly to fully black skin. Mold cultures may develop on the skin, and these should be thoroughly washed off when they become visible.

Hua Moa
Unmistakable appearance: fat and club-like with a blunt end. Possesses a deliciously sweet to sub-acid flavor.

Iholenes
Iholenes are tapered and have orange or orange-yellow peels. The eye-appealing orange pulp has a sub-acid flavor.

Berries

❖

Blackberry

•

Boysenberry

•

Loganberry

•

Blueberry

•

Cranberry

•

Currant

•

Gooseberry

•

Huckleberry

•

Jaboticaba

•

Limeberry

•

Mulberry

•

Raspberry

•

Strawberry

Berries

Common berries are native to Europe and North America. These aesthetically pleasing fruits grow from bushes, vines, or canes; and in the case of the strawberry, a plant. Cultivation has led to larger, juicier specimens with extended growing seasons.

Grow your own berries, buy from "u-pick" farms (preferably organically managed), or locate wild, unsprayed bushes, obtaining permission to pick where indicated. This ensures the highest quality with the added benefits of exercise and sunshine. Be sure to choose fully ripe berries because they will not ripen further once picked. Berry picking is an excellent chore for children, and can prove to be a valuable learning experience.

✎ Use the following *guidelines* at the market. Slightly firm, well-colored, dry, plump fruits indicate quality and freshness, while hard, off-colored ones are immature. Soft, watery specimens attest of rough handling. Shriveled or dull berries are past their prime. Avoid leaky fruits as evidenced by stickiness and stained cartons. Shun those that show the slightest sign of mold or decay. Obtain the cleanest berries possible so that they will not require vigorous washing, and therefore, fewer will be lost due to breakage—you save time and money.

Buy reasonably priced flats of peak-season berries and freeze or dry the surplus for year-round enjoyment.

Storage: Refrigerate those intended for fresh eating by placing them in shallow layers on trays or plates. This permits thorough air circulation, which in turn prevents early spoilage. Wash berries in cool water immediately before serving. A large bowl and colander are helpful.

Drying: Wash carefully and dry whole.

Freezing: Wash berries gently and transfer them into resealable freezer bags or plastic containers. To prevent breakage and bruising, lay bags on trays or baking sheets before placing the berries inside. Freeze and then remove the trays. Use fragile varieties within eight months. Blueberries, strawberries, and other hardy varieties keep for one year.

Blackberry *(Rubus nigrobaccus)*

Blackberries are the fruits of brambles—raspberries also share this distinction. Some blackberries grow on vines near the ground while others develop from vertical bushes. The tiny bubble-like structures that form blackberries (as well as raspberries and mulberries) are called "drupelets." In blackberries they appear as a collection of miniature black pearls that form a round to oval berry. Ripe blackberries are pitch black.

The dewberry *(Rubus trivialis)* is a blackberry that grows near the ground; hence the common name "running blackberry." Dewberries are smaller than common blackberries, and have larger, bluish-grey drupelets.
Season: May through September.
Nutrients: A good source for vitamin C, chlorine, and magnesium.
Class: Sub-acid

Boysenberry *(Rubus ursinus)*

A blackberry-loganberry-raspberry cross. Boysenberries appear to be oversized, elongated blackberries with burgundy to black drupelets. The original species are recommended over this hybrid.
Class: Sub-acid

Loganberry *(Rubus ursinus, loganobaccus)*

A blackberry-raspberry cross. Loganberries resemble elongated raspberries. Avoid and choose one of the original species.
Class: Acid

Blueberry *(Vaccinium corymbosum-highbush, V. angustifolium-lowbush)*

Blueberries grow on bushes belonging to the heath family. Cultivated varieties are classified as "highbush," while "wild" ones are called "lowbush." The cultivated berries are much larger than wild berries and grow on bushes 7 to 12 feet (2–4 m) high, allowing for easy machine harvesting. The result: enormous yields and reasonable prices. An incredible 125,000,000 pounds (57 million kg) of cultivated berries are produced in North America every year![12] This hasn't eliminated the gathering of wild berries which account for over 75,000,000 pounds (34 million kg) of the yearly harvest.[13]

Wild berries are smaller with the majority of the late July to August harvest being sold to manufacturing interests.[14]
Season: Purchase blueberries from April to September.

Buying: Look for large, powdery or silvery blue berries and use the general berry **guidelines**. The powdery sheen often seen on blueberries is called bloom, and indicates freshness. Bloom is the wax that God places on many fruits and vegetables to protect them from pests and the heat of the sun. Harvested berries lose their bloom in about one week's time. Darker coloring signifies lack of bloom, and therefore denotes aging. Instructions for storing, freezing, and drying can be found in the introduction at the beginning of the berry section.
Nutrients: A good source for vitamin C and iodine.
Class: Sub-acid

Cranberry *(Vaccinium macrocarpon)*

Cranberries are astringent fruits that grow on trailing vines. The plants thrive in low-lying bog lands that are flooded prior to harvesting. Machines agitate the vines causing berries to detach and float to the surface where they are easily gathered.

In the fresh state, cranberries are too bitter to be enjoyed; however, when dried they possess a pleasing tart-sweet flavor. Cranberries that have been processed in any other way are probably unfit for consumption due to cooking or the addition of refined sugars.
Buying: Firm, bright red berries indicate freshness.
Season: October to January.
Storage: Place in plastic containers or bags and refrigerate for up to three weeks.
Drying: Wash and dry whole.
Freezing: Wash, place in bags or containers, and freeze whole.
Nutrients: Extremely high in sulphur.
Class: Acid

Currant *(Ribes nigrum-black, R. rubrum-red, R. aureum-golden)*

Currants are small, smooth, round berries native to Western Europe. They grow in clusters from small bushes and share close relations with the gooseberry. Black, red, and white (or golden) species exist. Cultivation of black currants has

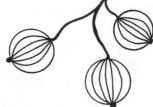

been prohibited in parts of North America because the bushes provide a breeding ground for a fungus responsible for disease among white-pine trees.[15]

White and red currants appear as little striped jewels—the work of an Artist. A limited number of varieties are suitable for fresh eating. Virtually all are processed into jams, jellies, and syrups; however, some of the white ones are quite sweet, possessing a flavor similar to green grapes.

Season: July and August.

Harvesting: To prevent bruising, pick the entire cluster.

Drying: Currants are commonly dried and have a deliciously tangy flavor.

Nutrients: An excellent source of vitamin C, potassium, and sulphur. Notable amounts of magnesium, phosphorus, and calcium.

Class: Acid

Gooseberry (Ribes grossularia-European, R. Hirtellum-N. American)

The gooseberry is a European native whose popularity in Great Britain has encouraged the cultivation of many sweet varieties that are suitable for fresh eating.

These round to oval berries grow on hardy shrubs and range from grape to egg-sized. Each is adorned in a beautiful shade of green, red, golden, or yellow, and masterfully designed with intricate, blood vessel-like striping. Sweet, fresh-eating varieties have thin skins.

Season: Summer and fall.

Nutrients: A good source for carotene and vitamin C.

Class: Acid

Huckleberry (Gaylussacia baccata)
Common Name: Whortleberry

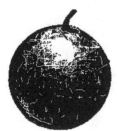

Huckleberry bushes are interesting because they can grow near the ground or reach 10 feet (3 m) in height. The bushes grow abundantly on the east coast (U.S.), and the berries are gathered from May to September. The tiny blue or black fruits are seeded and slightly sweet.

Nutrients: An excellent source for vitamin C and potassium.

Class: Sub-acid

Jaboticaba *(Myrciaria cauliflora)*

Jaboticabas are small, tree-grown berries native to Brazil. The dark blue, perfectly-round, white-fleshed berries are comparable in size to perlette grapes. Jaboticabas are tangy-sweet, although this flavor becomes overshadowed once the tart skin is thoroughly chewed. Overall, a pleasing combination.
Season: Summer
Buying: Not sold commercially.
Class: Acid

Limeberry *(Triphasia trifolia)*

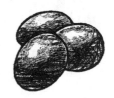

The exotic limeberry is a shrub-grown fruit native to India. These beautiful crimson berries are about the size of cherry pits and have a wonderful, tangy-tart flavor.
Buying: Unavailable in supermarkets.
Season: Summer
Class: Acid

Mulberry *(Morusalba-white, M. nigra-black, M. rubra-red)*

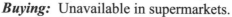

Native to China, the mulberry is a tree-grown berry that thrives in temperate climes. The elongated berries come in black, red, and white varieties, all of which possess a superb, tangy-sweet flavor.
Season: May through August.
Nutrients: High in vitamin C and potassium.
Class: Sub-acid

Raspberry *(Rubus idaeus-red, R. occidentalis-black, R. neglectus-purple)*

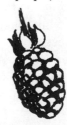

Although closely related to blackberries, raspberries differ because they develop around a receptacle. The result is a hollow, extremely fragile berry. Oddly enough, these highly perishable berries thrive in regions where the summer months

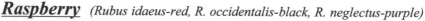

are cool and rainy. Red varieties are well-known but black and purple raspberries also exist. All types possess a delicious sub-acid flavor.
Season: June through October.
Nutrients: An excellent source for sulphur and chlorine. Significant amounts of vitamin C, niacin, potassium, and magnesium.
Class: Sub-acid

Strawberry (Fragaria chiloensis, F. virginiana)

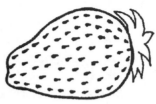

Native to North America and hardly needing description, strawberries are the most popular berries. Their appealing dark red color, fine flavor, availability, and easy growth throughout the continent has given them this distinction.

Strawberries belong to the rose family, but unlike other berries in this family, they grow on small plants near the ground. Secondly, the tiny seeds are embedded on the exterior of the fruit, giving them a "skinless" appearance.

The precursor of today's strawberry was developed in 1714 by crossing wild species from Virginia with one discovered in Chile.[16]

Most of our strawberries come from California. To increase production and fruit quality, California growers replant on a yearly basis.

☠ California growers also use huge amounts of carcinogenic chemicals on their fields. Strawberries have tender skins, preventing one from peeling or scrubbing off the outer pesticide residues. Look for a better source than supermarket berries or eat them sparingly.

✎ Home-growers: To stimulate optimal fruiting, pick strawberries as they become ripe.
Buying/Season: Select firm, glossy, deep red berries. Look for fresh green leaves, and avoid those that show signs of decay. The least expensive, highest-quality strawberries are available from April to June.
Storage: Strawberries oxidize quickly so cover them loosely with cellophane before refrigerating. Use within three days.
Serving: Organically grown berries need only be washed briefly, while supermarket berries should be washed with produce soap and warm water before being followed up by a cold rinse. To prevent water-logging, leave the caps on until the berries have been washed. Pluck the tops off with a "cap remover," knife, your fingers, or simply hold the leaves while eating.
Freezing: Strawberries lose their shape and firmness upon thawing. Minimize this effect by defrosting them in the refrigerator overnight. Use semi-frozen berries immediately.

Nutrients: An excellent source for vitamin C and silicon. Significant amounts of folic acid, potassium, and iodine.
Class: Acid

Black Sapote *(Diospyros digyna)*
Common Names: Chocolate pudding fruit, Black persimmon

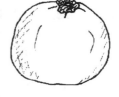

The black sapote is an exotic fruit common to Mexico. It is closely related to the Hachiya persimmon (see *Persimmon*) but differs in shape, having less uniformity and greater plumpness and size. The sapote's bright olive skin is about the thickness of a dime, and quite tough, requiring a sharp knife (preferably serrated) to easily slice it in half. The flesh appears black, but is dark brown, and has a gelatinous, pudding-like consistency; hence the name "chocolate pudding fruit." The flavor is mildly sweet.
Buying: Select ripe fruits (semisoft) or those just giving to pressure.
Storing: Once ripe, refrigerate for up to one week.
Serving: Halve and eat the pudding with a spoon.
Nutrients: Significant amounts of niacin and carotene.
Class: Sub-acid

Breadfruit *(Artocarpus communis)*

The exotic breadfruit is indigenous to India and the South Sea Islands. The bulbous, melon-sized fruits have olive green, honeycomb-designed skins. Upon ripening, the color becomes lighter and a pink cheek may develop. Once the fruit is harvested or drops to the ground it must be aged (ripened further). The belief that breadfruit requires cooking is a myth. An extremely soft, puckered fruit is evidence that the starches have been converted into sugars. Only at this point can the sweet, agreeable flavor be experienced. The seedless yellow flesh has a fibrous, creamy texture. Portions near the skin ripen first.

✎ When you think it is ready—wait at least several more days.
Buying: Select heavy fruits, and if possible, those that already yield to pressure.
Storing: Ripe, uncut breadfruit keeps for one to two weeks in the refrigerator.

Serving: Quarter and eat with a knife and fork, or slice vertically and spoon out the flesh.

Nutrients: An excellent source for B_1, vitamin C, and potassium. Significant amounts of sulphur, chlorine, iron, and calcium.

Class: Sweet

Cacao *(Theobroma cacao)*

Cacao pods grow on small trees indigenous to Tropical America. The trees produce sparingly, about twenty-five fruits per year. The pods are ridged, oblong to a point, and 6 to 12 inches (15-30 cm) in length. Immature fruits are dark green with variegated black striping, becoming light brown, yellow, or red when ready to harvest. Sweet-tasting, yellowish-ivory pulp surrounds the bitter beans that number 25 to 50 per pod. The *poisonous* beans are used to make chocolate.

☠ Chocolate and cocoa are outright health hazards due to the chemicals, contaminants, and additives they contain. The following information, as presented in the booklet *Poison With A Capital C*, is alarming and shocking, and should not be ignored.

The chemicals within chocolate are called methylxanthines. They can be further classified as theobromine, caffeine, and theophylline, all of which have deleterious effects on the body. Theobromine is known to cause a host of symptoms including abnormal glandular growth, nervousness, depression, anxiety, insomnia, gastrointestinal problems, and itching. Caffeine is highly suspected of being a carcinogen, and is directly linked to heart and circulatory problems, glandular difficulties, nervous disorders, osteoporosis, birthing abnormalities, and so forth. Theophylline causes stomach problems, nausea, vomiting, and nervous disorders.[17]

The processing of cacao beans into powder and chocolate is an unsanitary, risky procedure to say the least. To be blunt—*chocolate and cocoa are laced with animal feces and hair, insects, and molds*. The carcinogenic mold called aflatoxin has been found in large quantities on cacao beans![18]

Allowable limits have been set by the FDA regarding rodent feces and insect parts in chocolate and cocoa! As quoted from *Poison With a Capital C*, **"...every time you eat a chocolate bar, it may contain a rodent hair and 16 insect parts and still carry the blessing of the FDA.",** and **"For chocolate powder or cakes there must not be more than 75 insect fragments in three tablespoons of powder.",** and **"Four percent of cacao beans may be**

infested by insects. Animal excreta (such as visible rat droppings) must not exceed 10 milligrams per pound!".[19]

Chocolate and cocoa are unpalatable without the addition of refined sugars and milk. A great deal of scientific information has been published exposing the dangers of these two substances. Fresh and dried fruits constitute the sweets lovingly provided for man.

❑   *See Part 3 for deliciously sweet recipes, including milks, and **Carob** for a safe alternative to chocolate.*

The succulent, fleshy pulp of the cacao pod deserves a high rating, and should be experienced if obtained from a clean source.
Buying: Select well-colored, decay-free pods and age them until soft.
Storing: Ripe fruits should be refrigerated and used within two days.
Serving: Halve vertically, discard the seeds, and scoop the flesh out with a spoon, or quarter and eat with a fork.
Nutrients: An excellent source for vitamin C.
Class: Sweet (flesh)

Cactus Fruit (Opuntia stricta)
Common Names: Prickly pear, Indian fig

A native of Southern Florida, the cactus fruit is the offering of the Nopal cactus. Fruits are oval, 3 to 4 inches (8-10 cm) in length, and studded with barbs; hence the common name "prickly pear." Skin colors may be yellowish-green, crimson, or a tan-orange blend. Beneath the pliable skin lies sweet flesh riddled with hard, edible seeds. If it wasn't for the seeds, the cactus fruit would be a pleasure to eat.
Buying: Select those just giving to pressure and ripen them until soft.
Season: Peaks from August to December.
Storing: When ripe, cactus fruit may be refrigerated for up to one week.
Serving: Being careful to avoid the barbs, slice off both ends and score down the length of the skin before peeling it away. Cut into sections or eat out of hand.
Nutrients: A good source for vitamin C.
Class: Sub-acid

Caimito *(Chrysophyllum cainito)*
Common Name: Star apple

The caimito, a Tropical American native, is a round, green or purple, smooth-skinned fruit. Beneath its thick peel lies soft, jelled, white and pink flesh that possesses a delightfully sweet flavor. Two to five large seeds are situated inside.

Buying: Select large, heavy fruits with ultra-smooth skins.

Serving: When soft, slice horizontally to reveal a star design. Eat with a spoon, or quarter the fruit for out-of-hand enjoyment.

Class: Sweet

Canistel *(Lucuma nervosa)*
Common Name: Egg fruit

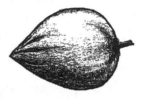

The canistel is a superb fruit indigenous to Central America. It grows from a tree of about 25 feet (8 m) and ripens during both the summer and winter months. Southern Florida also possesses a suitable growing climate.

Canistels are green when harvested and ripen to a mustard yellow within three to seven days. They have a very peculiar appearance, being round like an apple and smoothly tapering to a point from one to three inches long. The skins are thin and quite soft. This becomes apparent as they ripen, splitting wherever they please, generally from the point like the opening of a flower. The appearance and consistency of the golden flesh resembles the yolk of a hard-boiled egg; hence the common name "egg fruit." As many as four large, inedible seeds are imbedded in the flesh.

The canistel is a sweet satisfying meal in itself—one at a time is plenty! Due to its rich, throat-clogging texture, you must eat this fruit *very slowly*, savoring the experience.

Buying: Select firm, un-split fruits and ripen them at room temperature until soft.

Storing: When ripe, canistel may be kept for three to seven days in the refrigerator depending on the degree of splitting.

Serving: Break or slice open and eat with a spoon or a fork.

Freezing: Remove the seeds and scrape into freezer bags. Use within one year.

Nutrients: An outstanding source for vitamin C and niacin. Significant amounts of carotene.

Class: Sweet

Carissa Plum *(Carissa grandiflora)*

The carissa is a strange, shrub-produced fruit indigenous
to South Africa. This spherical, red plum is slightly
smaller than a walnut and contains soft, milky, pink
flesh. The "milk" is a form of latex that annoyingly sticks
to one's lips—and probably one's intestines, and therefore
heavy consumption is contraindicated. Several small, lentil-
like seeds reside within the pulp. The flavor is rather bland.
Buying: Not sold in supermarkets.
Class: Sub-acid

Carob *(Ceratonia siliqua)*
Common Names: St. John's bread, Honey locust

Carob trees are large pod-bearing
evergreens native to the Mediterranean.
The brown pods contain inedible seeds and a
pasty pulp, and grow up to 10 inches (25 cm) in
length.

The Scriptures tell us that carob was one of the principal dietary articles of
John the Baptist as he lived in the wilderness (…and his meat [food] was
locusts and wild honey. Matt. 3:4). "Locusts" was the term used to describe
the pods. Carob has been spoken of as "St. John's bread" up until this very day.

🌾 Carob is a delicious, naturally sweet fruit often used as a flavoring agent
to "substitute" the taste of chocolate; however, its flavor is superior to chocolate, and without the risks. Chocolate is bitter and only becomes edible when
laced with refined sugars and milk (See *Cacao* for more serious dangers).

*Carob has seventeen times less fat, three times the calcium, and one-third
the calories as compared to chocolate!*[20]
Buying: Carob is available in a number of forms including powder, chips,
pods, and syrup. Pure raw powder is the healthiest, safest, and most conven-
ient form. Order raw carob from health food stores or bulk natural food
distributors. Those who wish to locate natural food distributors can search
telephone directories or find out who supplies their local health food store.
Avoid carob products that contain sweeteners or dairy products.
Serving: Use for shakes, ice creams, sauces, toppings, pies, and any other
favorite recipes.
Storing: Pour powdered carob into glass jars or freezer bags and store in the
refrigerator for up to six months, or freeze for a year or more.
Nutrients: An excellent source for calcium, phosphorus, and protein.

☞ Carob contains significant amounts of tannin, which can bind protein, and therefore should not be fed to children on a daily basis.
Class: Sweet

Ceriman *(Monstera deliciosa)*

The ceriman is an exotic, beautiful plant indigenous to Mexico and Central America. Its stems climb from the soil to form wide-spreading, perforated leaves, and the peculiar fruits arise from the center and bear resemblance to Long English cucumbers standing on end (not shiny or smooth-skinned though). The ceriman's armor-like skin has been ingeniously designed into hundreds of pentagonal sections. These sections become increasing apparent as they separate and break away during the ripening process. Fruits are picked prior to this stage and left at room temperature. Patience is required because they ripen bit by bit over several days, starting from the stem end. One must eat the tender ivory pulp daily in proportion to the shedding of the outer layer. *Monstera deliciosa* truly lives up to its name: possessing a delightful aroma and wonderful pineapple-banana flavor.
Buying: Select fully intact fruits for freshness, sanitary reasons, and the avoidance of insect problems.
Season: Year-round.
Storing: Eat sections as they ripen, covering the end with a piece of cellophane and securing it with an elastic band to prevent the aforementioned difficulties.
Class: Sub-acid

Cherimoya *(Annona cherimola)*

The cherimoya is a delicious tree-grown fruit native to Peru and Ecuador. Its well-deserved popularity has encouraged an ever-growing commercial crop from California.

As a member of the annonaceous family, the cherimoya is closely related to the sugar apple and guanabana. Cherimoyas range from a pear to a pineapple in size and are generally heart-shaped but can differ greatly. Their olive green, leathery skins are etched in a teardrop design, while a gift of savory-sweet flesh lies beneath. The softly fibered granular flesh pulls away in sections, many of which contain tooth-sized, soft seeds that can number up to eighty per fruit. The flesh can be scraped right to the skin when the fruit is completely ripe. Cherimoya possess a delightful aroma and a not-soon-to-be-forgotten flavor.

Season: Year-round, peaking from July through October.

Buying: Cherimoya ripen off the tree if not harvested prematurely. Select fruits that do not have cuts or soft spots and ripen them at room temperature.

Serving: Ripe fruits yield easily to pressure and show separation around the stem. Halve them from the stem end to reveal the ivory or white flesh. Eat with a spoon, or quarter and use a knife and fork. Keep the seeds to grow.

Storing: Uncut ripe fruits will only last for two days in the refrigerator.

Freezing: Scrape the flesh into a bowl, remove the seeds, and place into freezer bags. Use within six months.

Nutrients: A good source for thiamine, riboflavin, niacin, and chlorine.

Class: Sub-acid

Cherry (Prunis avium)

The delicious cherry is one of the most sought-after fruits due to its fine, sweet flavor and limited season. Although native to China, cherries grow best on the west coast of North America. British Columbia, Washington, Oregon, Idaho, and Utah grow the majority of our cherries. Availability stretches from the second week in June till the middle of August.

These small, round to heart-shaped fruits grow in abundance from medium-sized, widespread trees, and require manual harvesting with the aid of ladders. The beauty of a cherry orchard should be experienced by everyone. Visit one (pesticide-free) for the sheer pleasure, freshest fruits, and lowest prices. Cherries do not develop further once picked, so gather fully mature fruits.

&⌢ Cherries are extremely vulnerable to rain during the final weeks preceding harvest—it causes them to split. Growers must take precautions to keep them dry during this period, before transferring the same responsibility to packers and consumers.

Buying: Cherries bruise and develop softness with the slightest mishandling, so be choosy—but careful. Select firm, plump, full-colored fruits that are free from splits. Green stems indicate freshness.

☠ Cherries often have higher pesticide residues that other fruits, and the skins are always eaten, so be sure to wash them thoroughly but gently (immediately before eating to prevent bruising) with warm water and produce soap.

Storing: Before refrigerating, spread cherries out on a plate or large tray to allow for thorough air circulation—dry cherries do not split. Fresh product in conjunction with prompt, proper refrigeration allows for a maximal storage time of two weeks. Follow with a cold rinse.

Drying: Wash, stem, halve, and pit the cherries. Place them skin-side-down and dry until a chewy, sticky consistency is reached.

Freezing: Wash tenderly, drain, and immediately set into resealable freezer bags (or shallow plastic containers), sucking out the excess air. To prevent bruising: position the bags on baking sheets, fill them, freeze, and then remove the trays. Cherries keep for eight months, but thaw mushy, so eat them while slightly frozen. Obviously, fresh cherries are far superior.

Nutrients: A good source for carotene, vitamin C, silicon, sulphur, and potassium.

Class: Sub-acid

Bings

The most widely cultivated variety due to their hardiness and outstanding sweet flavor. High quality Bings possess deep red to dark russet or almost black skins, and succulent, tender flesh. Available throughout cherry season.

Lamberts

Dark red, heart-shaped, and sweet. Lamberts arrive one week later than the Bings and finish up in August.

Rainiers

Aesthetically pleasing cherries with ivory to golden-blushed skins and clear, juicy flesh. Strikingly sweet. Unfortunately, limited production demands a heftier price. June through August.

Others

Van *(Bing x Lambert)* – hybrid, not recommended.
Royal Ann
Stella
Black Republican

Citrus

❖

Citron

•

Grapefruit

•

Kumquat

•

Lemon

•

Lime

•

Oranges

•

Temple Orange

•

Tangerines

•

Tangelos

•

Mandarins

•

Pummelo

•

Ugli

Citrus

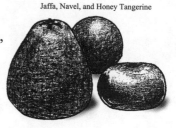

Jaffa, Navel, and Honey Tangerine

Citrus fruits have roots in South Asia, India, and the West Indies. Ponce de Leon brought orange seeds to Florida, resulting in the first trees by 1579.[21] Florida's perfect climate has enabled them to produce the majority of North America's needs.

The appearance and taste of citrus depends entirely upon growing conditions. For example, larger oranges are produced during warm, humid weather, while hot, dry conditions cause poor juice content. Cool evenings encourage better coloring;[22] however, the color generally has little to do with flavor. The sweetest oranges come to market later in the season (for each variety) and may be partially green due to substantial temperature changes. Brown scars or blemishes result from windy conditions and have no bearing on quality.

Buying: The demanding shopper feels the need to select the deepest colored oranges, but this temptation should be met with caution (especially in the early season) because handlers use dyes for artificial coloring.

☠ Citrus Red No. 2 is a food color that is used on the skins of oranges to increase eye-appeal, and therefore sales. This coloring produces cancer in animals[23]—and surely in humans as well. Of even greater concern is the fact that dyes assumed to be safe, prove to be lethal when combined.[24] Be sure that your children do not chew on the skins of citrus fruits (or other inedible-skinned fruits) because almost all of the colors, waxes, and pesticide residues are found on and in the peels.

    ❏   *Processed junk foods contain the largest amounts of food colors.*

🖉 Once harvested, citrus fruits will not develop further. Buy mid to late season within each variety and type. Stay clear of early-season, immature fruits because the acids they contain contribute to tooth enamel erosion.

As a rule, pick firm, heavy, smooth-skinned citrus. Firmness indicates freshness, heaviness signifies high juice content, and smooth skins mean more juice and fruit.

Storing: Citrus fruits must be kept cold to remain fresh. Product that was fresh when bought can be stored loose in the refrigerator for over one month (exceptions are listed).

Drying: Slice or peel, separate into sections, and dry.

Class: Acid

Citron *(Citrus medica)*

The citron is basically an oversized lemon with a rougher and much thicker rind. The rind is so thick that the remaining flesh is the lesser of the two. Not surprisingly, the flavor is sour. Citrons are produced for the rind which is candied or made into preserves.
Class: Acid

Grapefruit *(Citrus paradisi)*

The United States produces 55 to 60 percent of the world grapefruit market. About 80 percent of these come from Florida, with Texas, California, and Arizona accounting for the balance.[25] The highest quality grapefruits bear the Indian River label. These grow on the east coast of Florida.

Grapefruits vary in size as well as skin and flesh color. The Marsh variety has yellow skin and juicy, white, full-flavored flesh. It is classified as seedless, but usually contains a few seeds. Red grapefruits have pink to reddish flesh and yellow or pink skins. The Duncan is a larger, heavily-seeded fruit primarily used for juicing.
Nutrients: A good source for vitamin C and potassium.

Kumquat *(Fortunella crassifolia-sweet, F. japonica-round, F. arqarita-oval)*

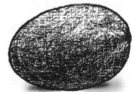

Kumquats are bite-sized orange fruits native to China. The three types, oval, sweet, and round, grow on small trees or shrubs. The oval and round varieties are sour. All three are said to have edible skins; however, the irritating oil within the skins will prove troublesome to the degree that it is ingested.
Season: Winter.
Buying: Select firm, deeply colored fruits.
Storing: Place into plastic containers or bags and keep for up to three weeks in the crisper.
Nutrients: Notable amounts of vitamin C, carotene, riboflavin, potassium, and calcium.
Class: Acid

Lemon *(Citrus limon)*

The sour lemon is native to South and Central America and
the United States. Most of our lemons come from California, Florida, Arizona, and Mexico.

✎ Lemons are prized for their sour flavor which results
from premature harvesting. The unconverted acids within
immature lemons have a deleterious effect on dental
enamel. Limes fall into the same category. Use both sparingly as flavoring
agents.

Season: Year-round. Less expensive during the winter.
Buying: Select firm, heavy lemons.
Class: Acid

Sweet Lemon

Some exotic lemons are mildly sweet. The *Limetta* falls into this category, and
appears to be an obese lemon.

Lime *(Citrus aurantifolia-Key, Mexican,*
W. Indian; C. latifolia-Persian, Tahiti)

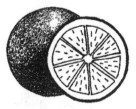

Common limes include the Persian or Tahiti
(actually native to California), and the Mexican.
Persian limes are larger with bright green skins
and light green flesh. Mexican limes and the Key
limes grown in Florida are small and entirely yellow
when mature.

Season: Year-round. Less expensive during the summer.
Buying: Select firm, heavy limes.
Class: Acid

Oranges *(Citrus sinensis)*

Orange trees reach heights of 30 feet (9 m) and are considered fully grown at
25 years. A mature tree can bear over 2000 oranges at once![26]

Sweet oranges are available year-round due to early and late varieties from
both Florida and California. For optimal quality, buy mid to late season within
each variety.

Hamlin
The first early-season Florida orange. Attractive, seedless, and thin-skinned, but lacks flavor and contains too much pulp. October to January. Bypass and choose late season California Valencias until January.

Pineapple
Florida's second arrival. Medium to large with a pebbly peel. Heavily seeded but very juicy and flavorful. A good choice for juicing or eating with a sharp knife, napkin, and plate. Available from November through March.

Navel
California's early-season offering. Small to extra-large with a thick, pebbly, peelable skin. Savory sweet. Available from November through June.

Valencia
Florida's finale. Medium to large and seedless with smooth, thin skins. Perhaps the best variety for juicing, and very nice for fresh eating. Availability stretches from March to August. Avoid early Valencias and choose California Navels until June.

California's late crop—May to December. The quality of California Valencias is poor, but they happen to be the only North American orange available in September and October. Sample some imports, or better yet, choose mangos, melons, berries, and other summer fruits. Buy California Valencias in November.

Jaffa
Large, thick-skinned oranges that elongate to the stem end. Jaffas have juicy, sweet flesh with very few seeds. Israel produces a substantial crop. Purchase from late winter to spring.

Blood
Blood oranges are small to medium with orange-red skin and sweet, softly textured red flesh. Available from winter to spring.

Nutrients: Sweet oranges, tangerines, and mandarins are excellent sources for vitamin C. They also contain significant amounts of calcium, potassium, and sulphur.

Bitter Oranges (Citrus auratium)

These large, bitter, heavily seeded oranges are processed into marmalade. The Seville is a well-known variety.

T–Fruit and Mandarins

Temple Orange *(Citrus sinensis x Citrus reticulata)*

A sweet orange-tangerine hybrid. Medium-sized, oval, and very easy to peel and segment. Since Temples are hybrids, the reader may wish to pass-them-up in favor of Tangerines, Navels, Valencias, and other sweet oranges.

Tangerines *(Citrus reticulata)*

Tangerines are characterized by good coloring, flat ends, seeds, and thin, peelable skins. The four common varieties include Robinson, Sunburst, Dancy, and Honey or Murcott. The first three have little flavor, but the Honey is superb. Its juicy, super-sweet flesh is the finest of all the citrus fruits. There are some seeds so be careful if you have small children. Honey tangerines are becoming reasonably priced as production increases. North American tangerines are available from February to April, while imports arrive in the summer.

Tangelos *(Citrus reticulata x Citrus grandis)*

Tangerine-pummelo hybrids. These small to large fruits have tight, deep orange-colored, difficult-to-peel skins. Seeded.

The Orlando (November-December) and the Minneola (December-January) are the two main varieties available in supermarkets. The Minneola is easily distinguished from other T-Fruits because it has a protruding stem, similar to the end of a lemon. Tangerines are preferable to tangelos since they have superior flavor and are non-hybrids.

Mandarins *(Citrus reticulata)*

Chinese and **Japanese** mandarins are imported during the early winter. Originally, only Japanese mandarins were seedless and superbly flavored; however, most of the Chinese oranges are now seedless, of superior flavor, and more reasonably priced. Seeded varieties of both types can be bought if so desired. Test the different brands because some are pulpy.

Prevent mold growth and extend the storage time (they do not last as long as other citrus fruits) by immediately transferring the oranges from their cardboard shipping boxes to the crisper. Before buying, check the box closely for signs of mold.

California mandarins are smaller and have a semi-tart to sweet flavor. The Satsuma is a common sweet variety.

Clementines are sweet, miniature mandarins imported from Spain and Morocco during the winter. Other imports arrive in the summer.

Pummelo *(Citrus grandis)*

Common Names: Shaddock, Pomelo, Pompelmous

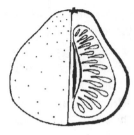

The pummelo, "grandfather to the grapefruit," holds the distinction of being the largest of all citrus fruits. Since the Pummelo is the precursor of the grapefruit, it is to be preferred. Pummelos grow well in subtropical locales, anywhere grapefruits thrive.

Pummelos have thick yellow skins that form a mound at the stem end. The segments may be yellow, amber, or different shades of pink. Unlike grapefruits, pummelos possess delicate, sweet flavors.

Buying: Select heavy, deep yellow fruits.
Season: November through March.
Storing: Store loose in the crisper for up to one month.
Nutrients: A wealthy source for vitamin C and potassium.
Class: Acid

Ugli *(Citrus reticulata x Citrus grandis)*

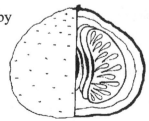

The ugli is a Jamaican fruit that was developed by crossing a pummelo with a tangerine. It looks like a small, slightly squashed pummelo but with thicker, loose-fitting, yellowish-orange skin. Since the Ugli is an overpriced hybrid, the reader is encouraged to avoid it, and to enjoy the less expensive original species.

Class: Acid

Coconut (*Cocos nucifera*)

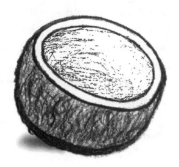

Coconuts grow from palm trees and are native to tropical climates. The sturdy palms not only supply an abundance of food, but furnish all the raw materials needed to create hats, baskets, mats, wreaths, and shelters. Coconut "meats" (edible white parts) and juice provide the makings for pure soaps, shampoos, and conditioners that possess unsurpassed moisturizing and cleansing qualities.

Coconuts grow near the palm's pinnacle just below the branches, and appear as huge, green or tanned in-shell filberts. A tough, fibrous husk surrounds the rock-hard nut. Three "eyes" are situated on each nut. Before cracking the nut open, use a hammer and ice pick to puncture two of the eyes, and then drain the delicious juice into a glass. Mature nuts contain *watery juice*, while young ones (picked green) have *creamy milk* because the fluid consists of the undeveloped meat in addition to the juice. Trimmed, young coconuts are "scalped" and sold as drinks in tropical countries. Some North American markets sell young coconuts.

The meat of a mature nut (copra) is about one half inch thick and tightly adheres to a tough, fibrous skin, which in turn is surrounded by the shell. Some suggest cooking the nut for easy removal of the meat, but this destroys or damages nutrients. To better complete this task, put the coconut (drained) into the freezer for at least one hour before cracking it open with a hammer. A sharp vegetable peeler can be used to pare off the skin.

Buying: Choose heavy nuts, indicating high juice content.

✎ Some handlers drain and refill coconuts prior to shipping: they use the juice and ship you water—hopefully clean. Inspect the "eyes" closely, making sure they have not been plugged with wax.

💣※ Avoid buying shredded coconut unless it is unsweetened and free from additives, preservatives, and fumigants. Fresh coconut is more flavorful and unoxidized.

Season: Year-round, but less expensive during the winter.

Storing: For peak flavor and lengthy storage, keep coconut in the freezer.

Nutrients: Magnesium, manganese, iron, and potassium predominate. Coconuts, almonds, and chestnuts are the only nuts that leave an alkaline ash upon metabolism.

🗁 Coconuts are high in saturated fat, but population groups that consume diets with a large percentage of their *fat calories* from coconut, fail to develop highly elevated levels of cholesterol.

Class: Protein

Date *(Phoenix dactylifera)*

Medjool, Barhi, and Halawi

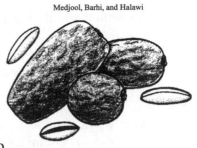

The date is an ancient fruit, probably given to man at creation. The Bible refers to the date palm a number of times: Exodus 15:27 describes seventy trees in E'-lim, the place where the Israelites camped after being led through the Red Sea by Moses. Jericho went by the name "city of palm trees."

Date palms grow abundantly in the Middle East, Africa, and closer to home, in California. They can attain lofty heights of 100 feet (30 m) and bear an incredible 600 pounds (272 kg) of fruit per year.[27] The dates grow in spectacular bundles, numbering up to 14 per tree, weighing as much as 40 pounds each, and sometimes containing a mind-boggling 1000 fruits![28]

Dates vary greatly in size and consistency. This is not surprising since there are over 7000 varieties in existence.[29] All types harbor a rock-hard, cylindrical pit. Fresh dates have smooth golden, brown, or reddish skins, and soft-to-chewy textures. Dried fruits are brown to russet, and chewy or firm.

Dates are the perfect foods to satisfy one's energy needs, and will easily extinguish cravings for unnatural sweets. Children should be given dates rather than candy.

Buying: At least nine varieties (11 types) are commercially available in North America. Supermarkets carry Deglets, Bread dates, and perhaps Medjools. These are non-organically grown, sulphured, fumigated, and possibly pasteurized. Those sold from bulk bins have been oiled or laced with other preservatives. Most health food stores stock organically grown or at least unsulphured Deglets, Bread dates, and Medjools, but examine them closely because some suppliers use oil as a preservative and for "ease in handling." For the greatest variety, freshest dates (organically grown), and lowest prices, order bulk quantities from a natural food distributor. To locate one who meets your needs, simply find out who supplies your local health food store or search the telephone directory.

Storing: For optimal flavor, keep dates in the freezer (up to one year). Due to their low moisture content, dates do not actually freeze; and therefore, few vitamins are destroyed. Dates can be warmed at room temperature in minutes.

Drying: Dry whole to desired consistency.

Nutrients: An outstanding source for iron, calcium, potassium, magnesium, chlorine, and all the B-complex vitamins.

Class: Sweet

Barhi
A superb date with dark coloring and a unique, sweet flavor.

Bread Dates
A dried Deglet. Dark brown appearance.

Deglet Noor
The most widely produced date—yet the least flavorful. Medium-sized and mildly sweet with a firm, semi-moist texture. Golden to tan skin.

Empress
A large, mouth-melting, sweet to extremely sweet date. The sweetness depends on the degree of sugar crystallization. Amber skin.

Halawi
A deliciously sweet date with soft flesh and golden skin. Mid-sized and reasonably priced, although the pits are often larger than other varieties.

Honey Dates
Honey dates are exceedingly sweet and possess a smooth, mouth-melting consistency. They ferment very quickly, so be sure to store them in the freezer. Thankfully, Honey dates are one of the least expensive varieties. The medium-sized fruits have thin amber skins.

Khadrawi
An extremely sweet, dark-skinned fruit with a soft, sticky consistency. Mid-sized and affordably priced.

Sugared Khadrawis
Khadrawi dates have invert sugar which crystallizes with aging, thus creating the tremendously sweet "sugared" khadrawi.

Lady Finger
A large, semi-moist date with little sweetness. Amber to light brown skin.

Medjool
A medium to extra-large, distinctively sweet date with a soft, dense texture. Medjools are unjustifiably expensive, especially since many of the other varieties have superior flavor.

Zahidi

A small to medium, firmly textured date with golden skin. The Zahidi has less sweetness than the other varieties, and not surprisingly, is the least expensive.

Durian (Durio zibethinus)

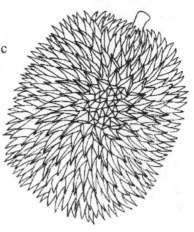

Indigenous to Southern Asia, the exotic durian is the most peculiar and dangerous of all fruits. These brown, ovoid, and often creased fruits are entirely arrayed with four to six-sided pyramidal spikes. The deadly spikes encourage the use of gloves when handling the fruit.

 Durians have caused serious injuries as they drop from their trees[30]—deaths have probably occurred since they often weigh over 20 pounds (9 kg)! Average fruits weigh 10 pounds.

The thick, tough rind is difficult to open, not just due to the spikes—but also the offensive odor of the flesh. A mix of onions, cheese, and rotten eggs closely describes the unpleasant aroma which diffuses through an entire house in a matter of minutes. The horrendous odor cannot be harnessed—even with several plastic bags!

Upon breaking open a durian, five substantial, vertical cavities become evident. The thick, fibrous rind extends to form these cavities which serve to mold the flesh into place. The off-yellow, softly fibered flesh is encased in a barely detectable transparent skin. The result: a creamy, slightly chewy texture. Onion-flavored cream cheese accurately depicts the savor, consistency, and aftertaste. If this flavor appeals to you, then you will love durian. Five large, shark fin-shaped seeds are mingled within the flesh of each cavity.

Buying: Many durians split, exposing the flesh before they ever reach the market. This is unhygienic, causes early decay, and allows the disagreeable odor to escape. Choose fully intact fruits, and if possible, those that are still cold or frozen. Durians are unreasonably priced in North America.

 To preserve freshness, handlers freeze durian before shipping; however, this may explain the occurrence of frequent splitting, because the fruit expands as it freezes and the rinds become easier to crack.

Storing: Eat immediately or store frozen.

Freezing: Place into plastic bags (because they can be disposed of), freeze, and use quickly.

Class: Sweet

Feijoa *(Feijoa sellowiana)*
Common Name: Pineapple guava

The feijoa is a shrub-grown fruit native to South America. Ours come from California in two harvests, spring and fall.

The ovoid, waxy green fruit is similar to a kiwi in size and a cucumber in feel. Slicing one in half reveals a beautiful kaleidoscope design, consisting of a gelatinous center surrounded by an ivory exterior. Tiny, edible seeds are dispersed throughout the jelly. The fragrant flesh is tart-sweet and somewhat gritty. A pineapple, strawberry, guava mix accurately describes the flavor.

Buying: Select plump, large fruits free from damage.

Storing: Ripen at room temperature until they yield easily to pressure. You must wait for full development or the taste will be very poor. When ready, keep for up to one week in the crisper.

Serving: Slice into rounds to reveal the beautiful design, halve and scoop out the flesh with a spoon, or eat with a knife and fork.

Drying: Dry as rounds.

Nutrients: Like the guava, high in vitamin C.

Class: Sub-acid

Fig *(Ficus carica)*

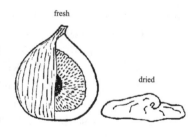

fresh

dried

Figs are among the finest, most delicious fruits given to man. Who can ignore that God provided figs for Adam and Eve in the Garden (Genesis 3:7). Surprisingly, these superb foods are relatively unknown or overlooked by most.

Figs grow on irregular, airy-branched trees. The fruits are bulbous and held by short stems. Immature figs are green, turning black, purple, or tan as they ripen. The edible skins serve as perfect receptacles, housing the jelly and providing an opening to accept a wasp—nature's perfectly designed pollination method for Calimyrna figs. The skins may be quite thick or appear to be melded with the flesh (as with fresh Black Missions) and the sweet jelly is riddled with tiny seeds. Commercially grown figs may be left to shrivel on the tree until they drop to the earth, followed by machine gathering, cleaning, and further sun-drying.

Figs can be eaten fresh but most are dried to preserve keeping qualities and maximize sweetness. Fresh figs have a fleshy consistency, while dried ones are chewy or firm. Only a small percentage of fresh figs reach the market due to rapid spoilage. There are generally two major harvests of fresh figs per year. Dried fruits are sweeter, less expensive, and available throughout the year.

Buying: Fresh figs must be clean, soft, plump, and free from breaks and decay. Eat them immediately or refrigerate and use within two days. Dried figs may be obtained from health food stores, but for larger quantities, order from a natural food distributor. To locate a distributor who meets your needs, search the telephone directory or simply find out who supplies your local health food store.

☠ Supermarket stringed, packaged, and bulk figs have been made unfit for consumption. Sulphur, potassium sorbate, oils, fumigants, and chemicals used in growing top the list of hazards (see *Dried Fruits* for more). Imports are always fumigated even though this is not required by law. Turkish imports have been found to contain extremely high levels of aflatoxin—a carcinogenic mold.[31]

᭟᭠ Figs (and other dried fruits) often develop a crusty or powdery sugar coating. These natural sugars accumulate due to temperature and humidity changes. "Sugaring" does not indicate spoilage but is merely a variation in appearance. Sugared fruits are tremendously sweet.

Storing: Place figs into jars or freezer bags and freeze for up to eighteen months. Refrigerate those for immediate use.

Serving: Soft dried figs can be eaten without presoaking.

✎ Soak firm fruits until the jelly rehydrates to a sticky consistency. This greatly eases digestion and improves the taste and texture. Place the desired amount of figs into a glass or bowl (stem-side-down) and cover generously with distilled water—distilled water is recommended so that the sweet soak water will be safe to drink or to use in recipes such as shakes. Set the glass of figs into the refrigerator and soak them until soft. This can take anywhere from 30 minutes to 12 hours depending on their firmness. Placing the figs stem-side-down prevents most of the sugar from seeping into the water, and refrigeration discourages bacterial growth, especially in hot weather or when the figs need to be soaked for a number of hours. Soak figs at room temperature for much quicker results. If you have insect problems then always use the refrigeration method.

Nutrients: Low-calorie dried figs are a tower-of-strength nutritionally speaking. Let us do a quick comparison between figs and milk, the so-called "perfect food"—milk is perfect, but only for the young (human or animal) as given by a healthy mother to her offspring until natural physiological changes indicate otherwise.

❑   *Comparison using 100 g portions.*

Milk (cow-WHOLE-3.7% fat)
Synopsis: 119 mg calcium, 100–110 mg potassium, and 0 g fiber. Excessively high in protein, fat, and calories, and lacking in iron. Milk has large amounts phosphorus, which lends to a poor calcium-to-phosphorus ratio. Contains exorbitant amounts of sodium and protein—high protein diets cause calcium to be leached from the bones and teeth (upsets acid-base balance). The calcium in cow's milk is difficult to obtain and largely unusable.[32, 33] Cow milk has been associated with a host of diseases including acne, allergies, anemia, multiple sclerosis, leukemia, cardiovascular diseases, kidney disease, asthma and other respiratory problems, diabetes, tooth decay [and osteoporosis], blood abnormalities, diarrhea, anti-social behavior, skin diseases, vomiting, and many others.[34, 35]

Figs (dried-uncooked)
Synopsis: 129 mg calcium, 640 mg potassium, 5.6 g fiber, 3 mg iron, and an excellent source for chlorine, silicon, sulphur, magnesium, and B vitamins. Very low in fat and calories. The highest alkaline-forming food available. All of the *organic* nutrients in raw figs, including the generous amounts of calcium, are readily available and easily assimilated.

The potassium content of figs is impressive—almost double the amount contained in bananas! Dried figs are an excellent source for iron, and have over 40 percent more fiber than raisin bran.[36]

❑   *Varieties listed in order of preference.*

Calimyrna
A superlative, tan-skinned fig with tremendous sweetness and satisfying jelled consistency. When fresh, the medium to large fruits are soft and tender skinned, and therefore may not require presoaking.

Black Mission
Black Missions have a distinctly sweet, rich flavor and a dense, chewy texture. The skins are black to dark purple and very thin (when fresh), appearing to be melded as one with the flesh. Black Missions can vary greatly in size.

Adriatic
A quality fig that closely resembles the Calimyrna but with less size and sweetness. Adriatics are generally stringed, and can be found in most markets during the fall and winter.

Kadota
A small, light-colored, thick-skinned fig with fewer seeds than the other varieties. Sold fresh or canned.

Grapes (Vitis vinifera, V. labrusca)

Grapes are ancient fruits thought to have originated in China, but like countless others, probably adorned the Garden of Eden. The Bible verifies that grapes have been produced for at least 3600 years. Grapes were eventually brought west in the 1700's by Spanish explorers,[37] and not surprisingly, quickly became a major food crop in California. At that time, the superb Muscat was the principle grape, but unfortunately, it has now been almost totally overshadowed by the many seedless varieties (see *Dried Fruits* for more).

Grapes grow in clusters from woody vines that often attain heights of 6 feet (2 m), and lengths of 100 feet (30 m) or more. They must be harvested manually and will not ripen once clipped from the vine.

Buying: Shop with a discriminating eye—freshness and maturity are the two keys. Do the grapes have full, distinct coloring? Is there decay, mold, or discoloration? Are they sticky or watery? Do they lack characteristic sizing? Are they starting to split, wrinkle, or separate from the stems? Do they feel soft, warm, and looked picked over? Are the stems green? Is there bloom—the natural wax that gradually disappears after harvesting?

A $1.00 per pound difference from week to week justifies buying extra grapes; however, it is pointless to bring home too many because optimal flavor with minimal loss is the goal.

❑ *Before reading the following, know that (on the whole) non-organically grown grapes (produce) contain fewer chemicals than animal products and processed junk foods, so eat with peace of mind taking the necessary precautions of course.*

Chemicals: One farmer, Paul Buxman, says that *seeded* grapes (and other fruits) are heartier and less susceptible to pests; and therefore, far fewer chemicals are used in production. He had to dispose of thirteen acres of rarely-sprayed seeded grapes simply because they would not sell. In contrast (he says), seedless varieties require spraying every five days throughout the growing season or they will rot.[38] This man has not used chemicals since the early 80's when his son was diagnosed with leukemia. Be aware that fungicides and sulphur are applied to almost all non-organically grown grapes. Sulphur cannot legally be used on fresh fruits and vegetables with the exception of grapes and potatoes. Dried fruits, although eaten raw, are also subjected to this hazardous treatment (see *Dried Fruits* for more).

Buy seeded grapes, and whenever possible, those that have been organically grown.

On a positive note, an *Associated Press* release from April 7, 1997 reported that purple grape juice contains a substance which is more effective than aspirin in preventing blood clots.[39] White grape juice also had beneficial properties. Be aware that acetylsalicylic acid has many serious and potentially fatal side effects, and these can be researched at any library.

Storage: Keep grapes in a cold, dry, oxygen deprived atmosphere—the refrigerator. Use within five to ten days depending on the variety, and cull (sort) them frequently to prevent mold growth and subsequent loss.

Follow these steps for extended storage: You need paper or cloth towels, plastic bags, and a suitable box. Line the box with two grocery bags and place one or two towels on the bottom to absorb moisture. Set several bunches inside and cover them with extra towels. Close the bags and refrigerate. Change wet towels during the daily culling. Dry towels can be reused if they have not been in contact with mold.

Serving: To remove exterior pesticide residues, non-organically grown grapes should be washed thoroughly with warm water and produce soap. For easier washing, you can clip grapes off their stems. Do not swallow grapes that taste strange.

Drying: Wash thoroughly and dry whole without preservatives.

Nutrients: All grapes contain a wide spectrum of vitamins and minerals, including vitamin C, potassium, carotene, and iron.

Class: Sub-acid

Muscat

The tangy-sweet Muscat is an ancient *seeded* grape that has probably been kept true to its original stock; and therefore, is recommended over all other varieties—refer to *Dried Fruits* for further elaboration.

Ribier

Delicious, juicy-fleshed blue berries. Round or oval, medium to extra-large, and *seeded*. Ribiers can be stored in the refrigerator for up to ten days. North American product is available from August to February, and Chilean supplies arrive during the winter.

Cape

An outstanding blue grape. Large to extra-large, nicely firm, and stores extremely well. The succulent, *seeded* flesh is pleasingly sweet. The Cape is a South African import that arrives during the winter.

Exotic

Large to extra-large blue berries that resemble Ribiers but with less flavor. *Seeded*. Marketed from June to August.

Emperor

Medium to large, oblong to oval berries with red blush. The flesh is firm, delicately sweet, and contains *seeds*. Few chemical problems. Long refrigerator life. Domestic fruits are available from September through March, and Chilean imports arrive for the winter.

Tokay

Large, *seeded*, red berries. Very tasty. Long storage life. Look for Tokays from August to November.

Queen

Delightfully-flavored, jumbo red berries. *Seeded*. Becoming increasingly available, and may be purchased from August to September.

Almeria

Large, oval, dusky-green berries with a fleshy texture and delicate taste. *Seeded*. October to February, but difficult to find.

Calmeria

Light green, elongated, semi-sweet berries. *Seeded*. Availability: October to February.

Concord/Corinth

Small, round, dark blue to black grapes with a tart-sweet flavor. Excellent if bought from a safe source. Tiny edible *seeds*. Domestic concords are available during September and October.

❑   Ruby Seedless, Cardinal, and Blue or Black Seedless grapes are not recommended since they are weak hybrids. Perlettes, Thompson Seedless, Red Flame, and all other seedless varieties may be hybrids too—further investigation is required—purchase seeded varieties whenever possible.

Guava *(Psidium guajava)*

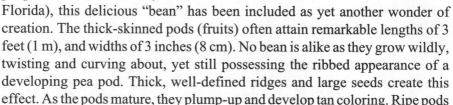

The Guava is an aromatic, highly irregular fruit common to Tropical America. The fruits can grow on shrubs or trees, appear round or pear-shaped, and vary from a cherry to an apple in size. Their skins are usually yellow but the flesh may be pink, yellow, ivory, or white. The gelatinous center is generously endowed with hard seeds, imparting an overall gritty texture. Savory flavors range from tart to tart-sweet. Guavas emit a definite musky fragrance that often justifies the question "what's that smell?" Fortunately, they ripen quickly.

Buying: Select those free from punctures and signs of insect infestation.
Storing: When soft, refrigerate for up to three days.
Serving: Halve and eat with a spoon.
Nutrients: An outstanding source of vitamin C. Significant amounts of carotene, niacin, potassium, and chlorine.
Class: Sub-acid

Inga *(Inga sp.)*
Common Name: Ice cream bean

The extremely rare Inga is indigenous to Tropical America. Although available to but a handful of people in North America (Southern Florida), this delicious "bean" has been included as yet another wonder of creation. The thick-skinned pods (fruits) often attain remarkable lengths of 3 feet (1 m), and widths of 3 inches (8 cm). No bean is alike as they grow wildly, twisting and curving about, yet still possessing the ribbed appearance of a developing pea pod. Thick, well-defined ridges and large seeds create this effect. As the pods mature, they plump-up and develop tan coloring. Ripe pods

are split open lengthwise to reveal white, spongy flesh whose superb flavor is reminiscent of watermelon. The seeds occupy much of the cavity.
Class: Sub-acid

Jakfruit (*Artocarpus heterophyllus*)

Native to India, the exotic jakfruit is easily the largest of all fruits—sometimes weighing over 110 pounds (50 kg)! The mammoth fruit has peculiar, green to yellowish knobby skin that resembles a foot massage mat. At a distance the Jakfruit appears to be a gluttonous, elongated breadfruit (a relative). Incredibly, jakfruit grow on the trunk of the tree—a sturdy tree. The heaviest, most sought after fruits arise from the roots.[40]

Buying: Jakfruit grow in Australia, Hawaii, Florida, and many tropical countries of the world. Select a yellowing fruit and wait for a disagreeable odor and deeper coloring.
Serving: Use a machete, ax, or large knife to sever the tough rind into lengthwise sections. The aromatic fleshy portions, arils (edible parts), are rich and savory-sweet like a mildly spiced banana. Remove the nut-like seeds—some people roast these.
Storage: Cover uneaten portions with cellophane, refrigerate, and use by the following day.
Drying: Since jakfruit are so large, it is practical to dry the fruit for future use. Cut the flesh into strips and dehydrate to desired consistency.
Freezing: Scoop the flesh into freezer bags or plastic containers, freeze, and use within six months.
Season: Year-round.
Nutrients: A good source for potassium.
Class: Sweet

Kiwano (*Cucurbitaceae member*)
Common Name: Horned melon

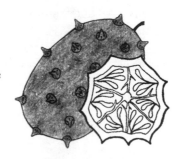

Kiwanos are native to New Zealand and have been placed in the cucumber family. These "horned" melons are easily distinguished by their bright orange, spiked skins. The oval to oblong fruits average 6 to 8 inches (15–20 cm) in length. Halving the fruit reveals a plenitude of cucumber-like seeds. A brilliant green jelly surrounds the seeds. The flavor and texture is said to resemble a heavily seeded cucumber touched with lemon juice.

💣 For those concerned, latest research has revealed the kiwano to be a "man-made" hybrid—an expensive one at that!
Class: Sub-acid vegetable-fruit

Kiwi (Actinidia chinensis)
Common Names: Yangtao, chinese gooseberry

The kiwi has rapidly gained popularity due to its delightful flavor and attractive appearance—once cut. This vine-grown fruit is native to China, but has really found a home in New Zealand where the finest kiwis now grow. California, Washington, and even British Columbia also grow kiwis. This allows for year-round availability: New Zealand fruits during the fall and winter, and North American product from late winter to fall.

The egg-shaped fruits have furry brown, paper-thin skins. An underlying green hue is often evident. Sliced width-wise, the kiwi displays its beauty in a brightly-colored jade, purple, and white starburst. The glistening, tangy-sweet flesh contains hundreds of miniature seeds. A soft, gritty texture and strawberry, pineapple, banana flavor lend to the kiwi's individuality.

Buying: Select large, plump, firm fruits and ripen at room temperature until they yield easily to pressure.

Storing: Refrigerate ripe kiwis for up to one week.

Serving: Halve and eat with a spoon, score lengthwise and peel the skin, or slice width-wise into thin, dazzlingly beautiful rounds.

Drying: Dry in wedges or rounds.

Freezing: Pare and quarter, or freeze whole. Use within six months.

Nutrients: An outstanding source for vitamin C and potassium. Significant amounts of vitamins E, B_6, and folic acid, as well as copper, magnesium, calcium, and iron.

Class: Acid

Litchi or Lychee *(Litchi chinensis)*

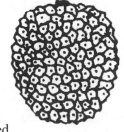

The succulent lychee is native to China and other subtropical to tropical locales. The walnut-sized fruits have an unusual outward appearance, characterized by a bumpy, abrasive, leathery skin. When harvested, the skins are dark pink, and remain so for four or five days before turning brown. The skins adhere tightly to the flesh, and when peeled, reveal the perfectly designed treasure inside. The glistening translucent flesh is juicy and super-sweet, and is ingeniously wrapped around a large, brown, inedible seed.

Season: Fresh lychees arrive during the summer and are only available for a few weeks.

Buying: Select large, firm, red-blushed fruits that are free from cracks, soft spots, and mold.

✎ Lychees are subject to worm infestation. To check for this problem, ask the retailer to peel one from the stem end: if you see a rusty discoloration or a tiny white worm—do not make the purchase.

Commercially, lychees are dried to make "nuts," canned whole, or processed into drinks. The drinks and canned fruits are laced with refined sugars.

Storing: Place fresh lychees in an airtight plastic container and refrigerate for up to three days.

Serving: Wash thoroughly with produce soap and warm water. Peel the skin (starting from the stem end), and carefully bite into the flesh so as to avoid the bitter-tasting seed.

Drying: Peel, unwrap the flesh from the seeds, and dry to a chewy consistency.

Freezing: Place unpeeled fruits into freezer bags or plastic containers. Freeze. Remove a desired portion and thaw in the refrigerator, or soak in warm water until the fruit yields to gentle pressure. Whichever method you choose, wash them well. Eat thawed lychees immediately, and use frozen ones within one year.

Nutrients: An excellent source for vitamin C. Significant amounts of potassium and phosphorus.

Class: Sweet to sub-acid

Diet By Design

Longan *(Euphoria longana)*

Common Name: Dragon's eyes

The longan is a small, round, exotic fruit that
is closely related to the lychee. It does not
match the lychee for beauty and sweetness,
but that's a tall order. Longans are grape-sized
and have thin, leathery, light brown skins. The
similarity to the lychee becomes evident after
the skin has been peeled away: revealing translucent, glistening flesh whose
tangy-sweet flavor is very satisfying.

Buying: Choose large, plump specimens free from mold, cracks, or signs of
decay. Follow the serving instructions for the lychee.

Season: July through October

Storage: Place in plastic containers and refrigerate for up to one week.

Drying: Peel, de-seed, and dry whole or in halves.

Freezing: Place into plastic containers or freezer bags and use within one
year.

Nutrients: A very good source for phosphorus and iron.

Class: Sub-acid

Loquat *(Eriobotrya japonica)*

Common Name: Japanese plum

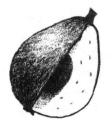

Loquats grow from small, productive trees native to China
and Japan. The fruits hang in clusters and vary from an
apricot to peach in size, shape, color, and skin texture.
The yellowish-orange flesh is juicy and tangy-sweet.
Three or four inedible seeds are situated inside. Treat as
you would an apricot.

Season: Fall and late winter.

Nutrients: An excellent source for potassium and carotene.

Class: Sub-acid

Mabolo *(Diospyros blancoi)*
Common Names: Velvet apple, peach bloom, scarlet fruit

The velvet apple is an interesting fruit indigenous to the Philippines. It appears to be an oversized, squat, red to russet peach, and has softly-textured, mildly sweet flesh. Select and treat as you would a peach.
Class: Sub-acid

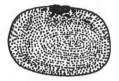

Mamey Sapote *(Pouteria sapota)*
Common Name: Mamey

The mamey is a sweet, satisfying fruit native to Central America. This peculiar specimen is oblong, coming to a point at one end, and varies from 5 to 10 inches (13–25 cm) in length and 3 to 5 inches (8–13 cm) in diameter. Severing the light brown, coarsely textured skin reveals russet colored flesh whose rich flavor and dense consistency is reminiscent of pumpkin pie. A large, elongated seed occupies the center.

᭡᭡ Prior to harvesting, the skins are scratched to determine the stage of maturity. If russet coloring is exposed then the fruit will ripen off the tree.
Buying: Mamey is available in Central America, other tropical locales, and in specialty fruit markets in the United States. Select semi-firm to firm fruits that have not been punctured or bruised.
Storing: Ripen at room temperature until they start to shrivel and become very soft. At this point they may be refrigerated for up to three days.
Serving: Halve from the stem end and scoop out the flesh with a spoon, or slice into wedges and eat with a fork.
Drying: Dry in strips to create sweet, chewy treats.
Freezing: Scrape the flesh into freezer bags or shallow plastic containers. Mamey freezes very well, lasting up to one year.
Nutrients: Notable amounts of carotene and vitamin C.
Class: Sweet

Mammea (Mammea americana)
Common Name: Mammea apple

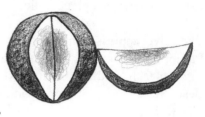

The mammea is an exotic tree-fruit indigenous to Tropical America. These brown, spherical, rough-skinned fruits vary from 4 to 8 inches (10–20 cm) in diameter, and possess soft, golden, apricot-flavored flesh. One to four large seeds are situated inside.

Buying: Available in Tropical countries and specialty fruit markets in the United States. Select firm or semisoft fruits and ripen until they yield to pressure.

Storing: When soft, refrigerate for up to one week.

Serving: Score and peel, or cut into wedges.

Class: Sub-acid to sweet

Mango (Mangifera indica)

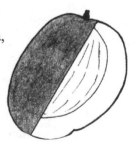

Mangos are luscious tropical fruits native to Asia, Mexico, and Tropical America. They have been cultivated for at least three thousand years and around 1700 were brought west to Brazil by Portuguese explorers. In 1889 a sea captain by the name of Haden planted Mulgoba seedlings in Florida.[41] This gave birth to the outstanding Haden mango whose savory sweetness surpasses all others. Southern Florida produces an ever-growing mango crop, although most of our supplies come from Mexico.

Mangos are aesthetically pleasing fruits of diverse shapes, sizes, colors, and flavors. Although classed as a sub-acid fruit, some varieties are extremely sweet. Upon ripening, the skins can display a rainbow of colors, while flesh tones vary from yellow to deep orange. A large, vertically situated, flat or semi-flat seed occupies much of the interior.

Buying: Mangos are at their peak when allowed to tree-ripen; however, they must be somewhat firm when commercially harvested to withstand transport. Those picked when simply mature enough to become soft will not develop full potential.

✐ Many mangos are improperly harvested by cutting the stem too close to the fruit. This causes "bleeding," the phenomena responsible for flesh-rot around the stem area, which in turn can quickly ruin the entire fruit. To reduce the chances of this happening, whenever possible, select mangos with at least a portion of the stem remaining. The Tommy Atkins is particularly vulnerable to post-harvest rot, in addition to being easily spoiled by the rigors of travel.

Sometimes mango seeds split and sprout, causing the surrounding flesh to become tainted. Tommy Atkins and Kent varieties often fall prey to this undesirable quality.

💣 Be careful when selecting mangos from a supermarket display, because when these fragile fruits are roughly handled, they will quickly spoil.

✎ Purchasing mangos by the case makes them affordable, and gives one the opportunity to select fully ripe, unbruised fruits.

Storing: Ripen mangos at room temperature, and for optimal flavor, only refrigerate those that have reached the height of perfection. Ripe fruits may be kept cold for up to one month, depending on the variety (see *Varieties* below).

Serving: One must eat mangos carefully since the juice stains clothing, table-cloths, and carpets. Some prefer to peel the skin and to use a knife and fork, while others will find the following technique the easiest.

You need a plate, spoon, and a small, high quality knife for precise maneuvering. Halve the mango by cutting down one side of the seed. Use a spoon to eat the flesh out of this half—this allows the flesh to be scraped right to the skin. With the second half, carefully score around the edge of the seed and slice underneath it from the front before lifting it out. Try not to slit any part of the skin to prevent juice from seeping onto the plate. Eat the flesh that clings to the seed, letting none go to waste, and then finish-up with the second half.

☐ *The recipe section describes a simple, decorative preparation method that only requires a sharp knife.*

Drying: Make two or three slices down each side of the mango, remove the peels, and dry as rounds or in strips. Be careful: thick pieces ferment. Dry or eat the remaining portions from around the seed.

Freezing: If you live in an area where mangos are cheaper than apples, than freezing becomes a viable option. As an occasional treat, use frozen mangos for shakes or ice creams, or better yet, simply thaw them until slightly cool and eat as a pudding. Preparation: Slice down each side of the seed and scrape the flesh from the halves and sides into a large bowl. Transfer to resealable freezer bags or plastic containers, and for convenience, freeze in ready-to-serve portions. Frozen mango can be kept for up to a full year.

Nutrients: Mangos contain more carotene than any other fresh fruit! Significant amounts of vitamin C, niacin, potassium, and chlorine.

Class: Sub-acid

Varieties

In North America we see five commonplace varieties that are dispersed from January to September. Winter imports are overpriced and often of poor quality. True "mango season" begins in April. Excellent, fair and poor shipments are unavoidable due to a wide range of factors including growing conditions, harvesting time and technique, transport, storage, and variations within the varieties.

Haden

Hadens are the first and generally the smallest of the common market mangos. Supplies start arriving in May but dwindle by mid June. A later harvest appears (in some supermarkets) at the end of July and lasts until September. Without question, the Haden is the sweetest mango. Perfect fruits possess succulent, slightly fibrous, deep orange flesh. The attractive skins display a rainbow of yellow, red, pink, and orange. Ripe Hadens yield easily to gentle pressure and emit a wonderful fruity aroma. When ripe, Hadens can be kept for a full month in the refrigerator. This allows one to buy larger quantities when the prices are low. At times, buying by the case can make mangos more economical than apples!

Tommy Atkins

The Tommy Atkins arrives in June and lasts until July, although in recent years supplies have flooded the market until August. This one deserves the lowest rating for taste, texture, and ripening qualities. It's inconsistent: small to melon-sized, smooth or stringy, tangy-sweet to poorly flavored, and keeps for one month or ferments before ever becoming ripe. Do not avoid the Tommy Atkins altogether, because some strains are excellent, and even the poorer ones are superior in flavor to many other fruits.

Kent

The Kent is a superb mango with fiberless, creamy-smooth to semi-resilient flesh. The fruits are generally mid-sized (but can get quite large), and may fail to attain deep golden color if harvested prematurely. Large black spots often develop on the skin. These spots will not affect the quality of the flesh if the fruit is not stored too long—trial and error. Ripe Kents can be stored for up to two weeks in the refrigerator (if the outer spots have not started to infringe upon the flesh). Available during July and early August.

Keitt

A late arrival in August, the Keitt (pronounced *kit*) is a tangy-sweet mango that can vary greatly in size. Ripe fruits generally remain slightly green so it is important to determine ripeness by feel, eating or refrigerating when they yield to gentle pressure. Keitts have a smaller seed in relation to their size. Regrettably, their season is very short, ending in September.

Francine, Oro
The Francine and Oro are deep yellow, kidney-shaped mangos that are usually imported from Haiti. The Oro is an unpredictable, overpriced, early variety, while the Francine arrives later and rates highly.

Carrie
The Carrie is a rare mango that is grown on a small scale in Southern Florida. It is small, fiberless, and deliciously sweet, and rates a close second to the Haden. The mouthwatering flesh possesses the consistency of an avocado.

Valentia Pride
A superlative, kidney-shaped mango with deep orange, delicately fibered flesh. The Valentia deserves to be rated third next to the Haden and Carrie. It is generally harvested twice during the summer.

Mangosteen *(Garcinia mangostana)*

The superb mangosteen is an exotic tree-grown fruit native to Indonesia. The orange-sized, reddish purple fruits have pepper-like stems and four cupped leaves that impart an overall rugged, yet attractive appearance. A tough, thick, pink rind encapsulates the snowy, sectioned, mouth-melting flesh, whose sweet flavor distinguishes the mangosteen as one of the finest of fruits.

Buying: Available in Asia, Tropical America, and specialty markets in North America. Select large, full-colored fruits.

Storing: Keep ripe mangosteens in the crisper for up to two weeks.

Serving: Use a sharp knife to make an incision around the circumference (being careful not to cut into the fleshy portions) so that the top can be easily removed.

Class: Sweet

Melons

Honeydew

•

Sharlyne

•

Crenshaw

•

Cantaloupe

•

Nutmeg

•

Casaba

•

Persian

•

Juan Canary

•

Watermelon

Melons

Melons are delicious, high-water-content fruits that are particularly satisfying during the hot summer months. They have been traced back to Eastern Asia and belong to the gourd family. The watermelon (cucumber family) has been classed as a vegetable, but because of its sweetness, most of us refer to it as a fruit.

❑   *Guidelines for buying and storing watermelons are discussed in detail under their own heading.*

Buying: Select fully ripe, heavy melons. Heavy fruits are chock-full of juice. Perfect melons yield to gentle pressure on the non-stem end and a reduced amount over the remainder of the surface. Thicker-skinned varieties do this to a lesser degree. Honeydews and crenshaws should be soft and "grab" one's hand as it is passed over the surface. Melons *do* bruise so handle them gently at the market, during transport, and at home.

💣※ Avoid overripe melons! Shake them: if you hear sloshing inside (especially honeydews) fermentation is well underway—poisonous alcohols have already formed and all the affected parts (perhaps the entire melon) would need to be discarded.

Melons can never ripen properly when harvested prematurely, so stay clear of immature fruits. They might get soft (or simply decay) but the sugar content remains virtually unchanged. Immature melons account for ninety-five percent of those available and are easily detected by their firmness, shiny-smooth texture (depending on variety), lack of characteristic coloring and fragrance, and chewy or hard, undesirably pale flesh. Melons should possess a clean, smooth break where the stem has separated from the vine. When melons are left to develop fully, the vine discontinues the food supply and then cleanly separates itself from the fruit. Jagged breaks indicate premature harvesting. Some varieties do ripen after being prematurely harvested, but can never reach their full potential. Larger fruits may be rotated to equalize sugar distribution.

🖋 For superior flavor and lower prices: choose watermelons, honeydews, and cantaloupes. Casabas are a welcome blessing in the fall. *Avoid out-of-season imports—they are outrageously priced and of poor quality.*

🖋 Buy whole melons because once cut, the flesh oxidizes very rapidly, causing nutrient loss and creating *free radicals*. Additionally, cut melon could be up to twenty times as expensive.

Storing: Whole, ripe melons can be refrigerated for up to seven days depending upon the variety and degree of ripeness (see varieties). Leftovers should be covered with cellophane, refrigerated immediately, and used as soon as possible.

Serving: Halve, scrape out the seeds and enjoy.

Drying: Dry in wedges, or blend and pour onto trays to make chewy leathers.

Nutrients: Outstanding sources for bromine. Significant amounts of vitamins C, E, and B-complex, as well as potassium, Cantaloupe and other orange-fleshed varieties are abundant in carotene.

Class: Neutral

> ❑ *The following melons (Cucumis melo) are listed in order of preference. The watermelon is discussed separately (at the end of the melon section) because it belongs to a different genus than the others.*

Honeydew

Without question, honeydews are the most luscious and savory of all melons. Vine-ripened fruits have tacky, light golden skin and succulent, ivory flesh. Perfect specimens are delightfully fragrant, and sweet and juicy right to the shell.

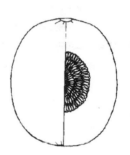

Orange-fleshed honeydews have deep orange flesh that penetrates the thin shell to impart an attractive orange glow. They are exceptionally flavored.

Season: Honeydews are available from March to October, but start buying in July.

Sharlyne

A succulent, sweet, ivory-fleshed melon whose fruity flavor rivals that of a honeydew. Sharlynes are golden (when ripe), lightly netted, and oblong, tapering to the stem on one end and widening at the other with an outward bulge on the bottom.

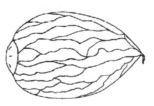

Crenshaw

The crenshaw has a unique shape, tapering sharply from the stem into an oblong, bulbous mass that forms a blunt end. They often get as large as

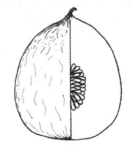

watermelons. Vine-ripened crenshaws are bright yellow to golden, and soft, with a tacky feel. Immature fruits are green. Perfect melons emit a fragrant, musky aroma and possess distinctively sweet, juicy flesh. Flesh colors may be yellow, ivory, or pink.

🖊 Slightly immature crenshaws do ripen well. Lay the melon on its side and turn once a day to equalize sugar distribution. Eat when it yields easily to gentle pressure.

Season: July to October

Cantaloupe

Cantaloupes as we see them in North American markets are really muskmelons. These are round, netted, and fragrant. Vine-ripened melons are juicy and delightfully flavored, but those picked too early (nearly all)—are worthless. Most "cantaloupe" varieties display an orange glow when fully mature.

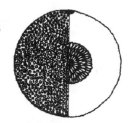

💣 Netted muskmelons are undoubtedly the worst keepers, readily showing age with mold and blackening in the stem's eye. You can detect these and other undesirable melons by their moldy odor, which indicates that the seeds and flesh have begun to decay.

Season: May through October—begin purchasing in June.

Nutmeg

The nutmeg closely resembles the cantaloupe (our market "cantaloupe") in most respects, but can be distinguished by its vertical grooving.

Season: July to October.

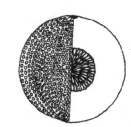

Casaba

Casabas are bright yellow, puckered melons of varying forms: Most are squat and wide, while others are oblong. They have juicy, ivory to pinkish flesh, whose delicate fruity flavor is a welcome change.

Season: Casabas have the benefit of a lengthy season, stretching from July through November.

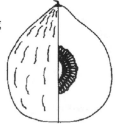

Persian

The Persian is a round, netted melon with green skin and orange flesh. This creates an attractive kaleidoscope design. Persians are delicious, but you can do better for flavor and price.
Season: June to October.

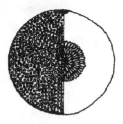

Juan Canary

Oblong and bright yellow in color, the Juan Canary is beautiful to look at; however, the ivory flesh more-often-than-not lacks sweetness. Some are very good, but why not buy less expensive, superior-flavored water-melons, cantaloupes, and honeydews?
Season: July to October.

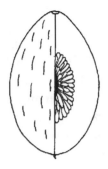

Watermelon (Citrullus vulgaris)

The succulent watermelon is an ancient fruit with roots in Asia and Africa. The Bible records watermelons as being grown as far back as ancient Egypt (Numbers 11:5). Archeologists have substantiated the Scriptures by finding watermelon drawings in many Egyptian tombs.

Watermelons differ from other melons in that they do not have a seed-containing cavity—the flesh reaches from one end to the other and is housed by a thick rind. Larger melons may have a hollow spot.

Most of our watermelons come from Texas, Georgia, and California. With over fifty varieties, one can expect them to vary in size, shape, and color. Small "ice-box" melons weigh as little as 5 pounds (2.3 kg), while fruits of 15 pounds or more are classified as "picnic." The largest one on record weighed a whopping 255 pounds (116 kg)![42] Seedless and yellow-fleshed varieties exist.
Buying: No one can guarantee a perfect watermelon, but the following tips will greatly improve your chances of selecting one that is fresh and sweet. Larger melons are generally sweeter. Choose those with yellow or white underbellies, indicating a lengthy time on the ground. Superb melons possess

deep, fully-colored flesh with a small number of firm, dark seeds and a minimal amount of white fibrous tissue. The flesh should be juicy and bursting with flavor. Poor melons have rubbery, flavorless flesh which lacks juice, sheen, and crispness.

Can slapping, thumping, or knocking provide a clue for selecting an excellent melon? Possibly, but the fruit must be fresh (very firm, even on the ends). This being the case, large, oval to round melons should sound full and "dead," while oblong and smaller fruits may have a clear, crisp reverberation.

💣 Watermelons are fragile and easily damaged by tossing and overpiling—this is one reason for soft melons at the market; others include age and poor storage. Resist the temptation to buy those that yield easily to pressure because fermentation is well underway.

Buy whole melons because cut fruits are costly, oxidized, and serve as yet another source of chemical exposure because the cellophane is in contact with high percentages of the flesh for lengthy periods of time.

🖉 At the market, examine the cut watermelons to see whether the whole ones are worth buying.

A Better Choice: Test results consistently show domestic watermelons to contain low levels of pesticides—definitely one of the safest choices for you and your children.

Season: April through October, peaking from June to August.

Storing: Always refrigerate cut melons, and whole ones whenever possible. Cut fruits that have but one surface of the flesh exposed should be consumed within three days, while portions with more exposure need to used within 24 hours. Fresh whole melons should be kept cool and used before the ends become soft.

Serving: Cut into horizontal slices from one end (as needed) to reduce the amount of exposed flesh on leftovers. Quickly cover the uneaten portion with cellophane and refrigerate.

Nutrients: Watermelon is the highest raw food source of bromine known to man! An apple has 0.15 mg of bromine per 100 g edible portion, while the watermelon has 26.20 milligrams.[43] Watermelons are also rich in vitamins C, E, the entire B-complex, and carotene, as well as potassium, magnesium, and iron.

Crimson Sweet

A high quality melon that deserves to be rated first or second. Round to slightly oval with a light green base and variegated, dark green striping. Deep red flesh. Weights generally vary from 15 to 35 pounds (7–16 kg).

Allsweet
Could be your favorite, and at its best is the sweetest. Oblong with a light to medium green base and dark green stripes. Dark red flesh. Allsweets can reach mammoth weights of 40 pounds (18 kg) or more.

Jubilee
Oblong with a light green base and variegated, dark green stripes. Medium red flesh. Rivals the Allsweet for size, often exceeding the 40 pound (18 kg) mark.

Charleston Grey
Oblong with a blood vessel-designed, light green rind. Deep red flesh. Weights range from 15 to 35 pounds (7–16 kg).

Peacock/Calsweet
Oval to oblong with a dark green rind and red flesh. The flesh of the Peacock is often quite fibrous so be sure that the source is good before buying a large quantity. They commonly weigh from 15 to 25 pounds (7–11 kg).

Ice-box
Small, round fruits with light to dark green rinds and red or yellow flesh. Ice-box melons are generally under 15 pounds (7kg).

Yellowflesh
Assorted sizes and shapes with variegated dark green stripes. Less sweet. Average melons weigh from 20 to 25 pounds (9–11 kg).

Seedless
Round to oval with dark green stripes. Red or yellow flesh. Weights are generally under 25 pounds (11 kg).

🖋 Fewer pesticides are used on seeded varieties, which also happen to possess superior flavor. Seedless varieties are probably hybrids.

Mombin *(Spondias mombin)*

Mombins are large, delicious, fragrant berries native to Tropical America. They grow from wild, wide-spreading trees of about 25 feet (8 m). The prolific trees bear thousands of green, kumquat-sized berries, each of which ripens gradually, turning pale yellow before developing brilliant red to crimson tones. Thankfully, this does not happen

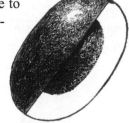

overnight. It takes three months for all the berries to mature. A tree displaying ripe mombins is a beautiful, not-soon-to-be-forgotten sight. Yellow and breathtaking purple varieties also exist.

Mombins possess a wonderful fruity aroma. The savory golden flesh is tangy and very juicy, while the skins add chewiness. A large oblong seed occupies nearly half of this very fragile berry.

Buying: Not available in supermarkets.

Class: Sub-acid

Nectarine *(Prunus persica)*

Mistakenly thought to be a cross between a peach and a plum, the nectarine is truly a distinct fruit, dating back at least 2000 years to Asia. They do appear to be fuzzless peaches and grow from a similar tree.

Nectarines have smooth, creased skins with yellow base coloring and red blush. The golden to golden-red flesh is succulent and tangy-sweet—superior to that of the peach. Freestone and semi-clingstone varieties exist.

Season: May through September.

Buying: Select firm, full-colored fruits. Check the stem area, avoiding those tinged with green or showing signs of interior decay.

●※ Shun the South American imports that arrive during our winter months because they are picked prematurely, have dry, woody flesh, and are prone to flesh rot (spoilage that starts from around the stone).

Storing: Refrigerate ripe nectarines for up to two weeks. To prevent bruising, place them on a plate or suitable flat surface.

Drying: Slice into wedges and dry until chewy.

Freezing: Freeze in halves or quarters and use within one year.

Nutrients: An outstanding source for carotene. Significant amounts of potassium and vitamins C, folic acid, and B$_2$.

Class: Sub-acid

Flavortop
Tangy-sweet smooth flesh. Select those with three-fourths red blush. July through August.

Fantasia
Superlative sweet flavor. Should display three-fourths red blush. July through August.

Red Gold
Full-colored and sweet. August through September.

Olive (Olea europaea)

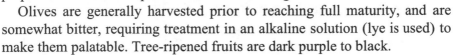

Being an ancient fruit, the olive is native to Asia, and has been cultivated extensively for over 3000 years. To this day they remain a major commercial crop with Italy, Spain, Greece, and Portugal topping the list of producers. In the days that Jesus walked this earth, olive oil was used in cooking, lamps, ointments, and hair rinses, while the pulp was made into soaps and served as kindling for fires.[44]

Olives are generally harvested prior to reaching full maturity, and are somewhat bitter, requiring treatment in an alkaline solution (lye is used) to make them palatable. Tree-ripened fruits are dark purple to black.

☧ Olives are an excellent food, but modern-day processing techniques *may be* as follows: olives are fermented in lactic acid, artificially colored, and treated with lye before being packed in a salt solution.[45] During these processes the natural sugars are destroyed, while alcohols and lactic and acetic acids remain[46]—Acetic acid happens to be one of the harmful breakdown products of alcohol (the commonly sold poison), and this is one of the reasons why vinegar (generally five percent acetic acid, and used in condiments etc.) has a damaging effect upon the body. Some olive processors add carrageenan, which is thought to play a role in colitis and genetic alterations.[47] Other additives or preservatives are also commonly used so check labels and either avoid the olives altogether or soak them in pure water and rinse thoroughly.
Buying: Search until an acceptable brand is found. You may have to visit a specialty market, buy from a bulk food distributor, or purchase large cans to avoid undesirable additives and preservatives. Whenever possible, use whole olives.

✒ Even those olives that have not been subjected to the worst treatments will contain excessive amounts of salt, and therefore pose a health risk to those on low-sodium diets. To remove most of the salt, soak them in pure water and rinse thoroughly.
Nutrients: High in iron.
Class: Protein-fat

Papaya *(Carica papaya)*

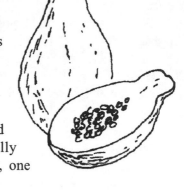

Oddly enough, the prolific papaya plant has been classed as a giant herb.[48] It appears to be a palm tree with the leaves sprouting from the trunk, and can reach heights of over 20 feet (6 m) yet still have a diameter of under 8 inches (20 cm). The fruits, surprisingly called berries,[49] grow from short stems generally located near the top of the plant. To pick, one simply twists the fruit.

Many varieties of papaya exist as evidenced by the wide range of sizes, shapes, colors, and flavors. Common supermarket fruits are small and pear-shaped. Remarkably, papayas can weigh from $\frac{1}{2}$ to 20 pounds (0.22–9 kg). Upon ripening, the thin green skins become yellow or orange, while the creamy-smooth flesh possesses deeper coloring and may be muddy yellow, pink, or red. Small, wrinkled black seeds line the sides of the inner cavity. These *inedible* seeds are encapsulated by fluid-filled sacs.

Hawaiian-grown papayas are superior to all others. Island varieties include Solo, Kuuku, and Strawberry (Sunrise). The Solo is the most common type and can be found throughout Hawaii as well as on the mainland. Kuukus are rarely seen, more expensive, and have deeper flesh color. Their delicious flavor is richer and sweeter than the Solo. Strawberry papayas are also less common and more costly. Their attractive dark pink to reddish flesh is responsible for the name (outwardly appear to be Solos). The Strawberry papaya is the juiciest and sweetest variety, and has a mouth-melting consistency similar to a ripe honeydew. When fully ripe, the savory flesh can be scraped right to the papery thin skin.

Season: Year-round, peaking from October to December, and April through July.

Buying: Select unbruised, fragrant fruits with at least 50 percent yellow coloring. *Handle gently!*

✐ Check directly around the stem: if there is a yellow hue then it will ripen properly.

Storage: Ripen at room temperature. Color cannot be relied upon as a gauge for ripeness if you select prematurely harvested fruits. Judge by feel unless it is apparent that color will be a reliable guide. Perfect papayas are fragrant, entirely yellow, and yield easily to pressure. At this point they can be refrigerated for one week or more.

Serving: Halve lengthwise, scrape out the seeds, and eat with a spoon, or slice into wedges and use a knife and fork.

Drying: Slice into quarter inch strips, remove the skin, and dehydrate until firm.

Freezing: Scoop the flesh into resealable freezer bags or shallow plastic containers, freeze, and use within six months.

Nutrients: An outstanding source for carotene and vitamin C. Significant amounts of potassium.

📂 Papayas contain an enzyme called papain which is similar to the protein-digesting enzyme pepsin, which is secreted into the human stomach. The digestion of nuts is noticeably improved when papaya has formed part of the meal or the day's diet. Papayas contain large amounts of soft fiber, and this lends to a rapid transit time. Therefore, papayas are perfect for those with digestive and intestinal disorders as well as all who wish to remain healthy.

Class: Sub-acid

Passion Fruit *(Passiflora edulis)*

Native to Brazil, the passion fruit is a vine-grown delicacy whose unappetizing appearance is but skin deep. Upon ripening, passion fruit develop a dimpled complexion, and if one did not know better, would toss the unappetizing specimens into the trash. The egg-shaped fruits attain lengths of three inches (8 cm) and have tough, purple or yellow skins. The edible portion consists of yellow juice, seeds, and membranous tangy-tart flesh.

Buying: Choose heavy, deeply colored fruits. Unripe passion fruits ripen within two to five days.

Storing: Keep ripe ones in the crisper for up to one week.

Serving: Halve and eat right from the shell with a spoon, or scrape into a bowl or on top of other fruits.

Freezing: Passion fruit freezes extremely well, lasting up to one year. Wash, dry, and place into freezer bags or plastic containers. Thaw overnight in the refrigerator.

Nutrients: An excellent source for vitamin C, carotene, niacin, potassium, and iron.

Class: Acid

Pawpaw (Asimina triloba)

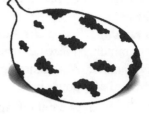

Although frequently confused with the papaya, the pawpaw is an entirely different fruit. This United States native grows from a small to medium, thin-branched tree that can produce fruit throughout the year, although most frequently during the late summer and early fall. The fruits have the appearance of short, stubby bananas that have been pumped full of air to the point of bursting. Dark markings develop as they mature. Severing the skin reveals the fragrant yellow flesh whose flavor can be likened to a blend of banana, pineapple, and papaya. Several large, black, inedible seeds are embedded within the flesh.

Buying: Pawpaws grow wild along riverbeds and in valleys in isolated regions of the central and southern states. Ripe fruits yield easily to pressure.

Serving: Halve lengthwise and spoon out the flesh.

Nutrients: Few nutritional statistics exist on the pawpaw. *Composition and Facts About Foods* lists the pawpaw as being higher in protein than all fresh and dried fruits. A 100 g portion has 5.2 g of protein. To put this in perspective, the orange contains 1 g, the banana 1.1 g, and dried figs 4.3 grams.[50]

Class: Sub-acid

Peach (Prunus persica)

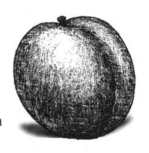

Peaches are ancient stone fruits native to China. These fuzzy, spherical to heart-shaped fruits are distinctively creased and possess varying degrees of blush. Their tender skins yield to sweet, succulent golden flesh that is often splashed with a red starburst which originates from the center. Freestone and semi-clingstone varieties exist.

Buying: Peaches are the most delicate and perishable stone fruits due to their size, fragile skin, and supple flesh. Select firm peaches that are free from bruises and skin damage. Look for those with a definite crease and full coloring, being sure to examine the stem area for tinges of green (indicating immaturity) or signs of interior decay.

✎ Take a box to transport your investment.

The most flavorful market varieties include Flavorcrest, Regina, Red Haven, and the June, Summer, Scarlet and Elegant Ladies.

💣⃰ Avoid out of season imports.

Season: June through September.
Storing: Ripen at room temperature. To prevent bruising, place ripe fruits on a plate or suitable flat surface before transferring into the refrigerator. Keep for up to four days.
Drying: Dry in wedges or slices to desired consistency.
Freezing: Wash, quarter, and set (single-layer-high) into freezer bags, or place into shallow plastic containers. Lay flat until frozen and use within one year.
Nutrients: Substantial quantities of carotene. A good source for potassium, sulfur, niacin, and vitamin C.
Class: Sub-acid

Forelle

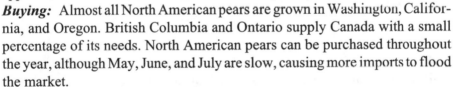

Pears (Pyrus communis)

Ancient fruits, pears date back at least 3000 years to Asia. Of the 3000 varieties only eight or nine are grown extensively.[51]

Pear trees can attain heights of 45 feet (14 m), and possess impressive spans of 25 feet (8 m).[52] They frequently reach 100 years, doubling the lifespan of an apple tree.[53] Dwarf trees are under 8 feet tall (2.4 m).

Buying: Almost all North American pears are grown in Washington, California, and Oregon. British Columbia and Ontario supply Canada with a small percentage of its needs. North American pears can be purchased throughout the year, although May, June, and July are slow, causing more imports to flood the market.

Pears must be harvested when firm. Those picked late ripen mushy, while premature fruits develop dry, spongy, flavorless flesh. Avoid the first crops from all varieties.

✐ Select firm, undamaged fruits just breaking in color to ensure complete ripening.
Storing: Ripen at room temperature, always using feel to determine ripeness. Pears are ready when the area around the stem yields easily to gentle pressure. At this point they should emit a wonderful fragrance. When ready, keep for up to several days in the refrigerator (see each variety for keeping qualities).
Nutrients: A very good source for vitamins E, C, B$_2$, and folic acid, as well as potassium and magnesium.
Class: Sub-acid

❏   *Varieties listed alphabetically.*

Anjou

Anjous are sweet, juicy, fine to medium-textured pears native
to Belgium. They have smooth skins and a rounded,
"no-neck" appearance. Those that have not been harvested
prematurely develop light green to yellow coloring.

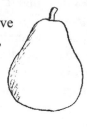

Advantages include outstanding storage qualities,
unique flavor, reasonable prices, and availability during
the scarce "pear months" (March to June). Washington
produces fantastic, oversized Anjous.

Red Anjous are becoming increasingly available, but choose the originals
for better flavor and price.

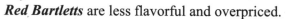

Bartlett

The consumer's choice. Fully ripe Barletts possess juicy,
delightfully fragrant, sweet flesh and attractive yellow
skins which often display a pink cheek. At their best,
Barletts rate along side the Bosc, Comice, and
Florelle. The Bartlett is the only pear considered to
be a summer fruit. They arrive in July and last until
December with the aid of cold storage. Superior
during August and September. Once ripe they store
poorly.

Red Bartletts are less flavorful and overpriced.

Bosc

A succulent, savory pear native to Belgium. The Bosc has an
unmistakable appearance, characterized by a long tapered
neck and tan to dark brown skin. High quality fruits possess a
superb flavor that surpasses all other varieties. Boscs are
less susceptible to bruising, and when ripe, can be kept for
up to one week in the refrigerator. North American fruits
(August to May) are superior from September through
December.

Comice

Thought to have originated in France, the Comice is perhaps the
sweetest and juiciest of all pears. The small to large, luscious
fruits are yellowish-green and often adorned with a pink
cheek. Little if any neck definition is evident. Their delicate
skins frequently show wind scars but these have no bearing
on quality. Available from September through December.

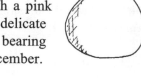

Forelle
A small pear, similar in shape to the Bartlett but with less neck definition. Upon ripening, the green, red-freckled skins transform to yellow (or yellowish-green) and bright red. The succulent flesh possesses a unique, spicy-sweet flavor, thus giving the Florelle the distinction of being one of the finest of pears. Availability stretches from September through February.

Nelis
A mid-sized, stubby pear with a rounded appearance. The light green skins (most often becoming yellow) are marbled with brown, and the flesh is smoothly textured and pleasantly sweet. Available from October to May, but difficult to find in many regions.

Packham Triumph
Resembles the Bartlett but with less flavor. Available as an import during our slower pear months.

Seckel
The Seckel is the short, stubby pear with olive-green and burgundy skin. It possesses a distinctively sweet flavor. Select those that display a high degree of blush. Available from September to December.

Persimmon (Diospyros kaki - Japanese, D. virginiana - American)
Common names: Kaki, Date plum

Persimmons are among the sweetest, most satisfying fruits given to man. In the Orient they are known as kaki or date plums.

    Japanese persimmons can be divided into three types according to their degree of softness when ripe: firm, semi-soft, and very soft.

Soft-When-Ripe
The Hachiya is the most common soft-when-ripe variety. It looks like a conical or acorn-shaped orange tomato and has paper-thin, membranous skin, making it extremely fragile as it ripens. The flesh is light to deep orange and contains up to eight elliptic, dark seeds. Most are seedless with the odd one containing one or two seeds.

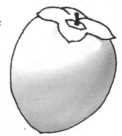

Buying: Select soft to firm, deep orange or red Hachiyas that are free from mold. Avoid rock-hard, poorly colored persimmons because they will never ripen properly. If you decide to buy those that are fully ripe, be sure that they have not been bruised or punctured.

Purchase persimmons by the flat, or take empty boxes with you for loading those that are displayed individually. Flats are usually less expensive.

A Better Choice: Persimmons are highly resistant to pests, so many commercial growers do not use pesticides. Look for certified organically grown stickers.

Storing: Once ripe, refrigerate for up to four days.

✏ As persimmons ripen, mold and decay are prone to occur around the stem and under the leaves. Examine these areas before making a purchase, and once home, tear away the outer leaves as soon as possible (before the fruits become soft). This prevents spoilage and guards against punctures caused by the leaves which become dry and jagged. It also simplifies washing and eating.

✏ A fully ripe Hachiya feels like a water-filled plastic bag. All soft-when-ripe persimmons are astringent until this point, and impatience results in an unpleasant taste experience. The astringency is due to tannin which must be given the opportunity to crystalize.[54] When you think it is ready, wait a day or two.

Serving: Rest the stem end in your palm and gently bite into the tip, sucking out the juice and flesh; or place on a plate or in a bowl, remove the stem, and eat with a knife and spoon.

Drying: Cut into slices and dry to desired consistency.

Freezing: Freezing unripe persimmons crystallizes most of the tannin. Upon thawing, the astringency has disappeared; however, natural ripening at room temperature is preferable because it allows the nutrients to develop completely.

Wash, dry, and place fruits (leaves already removed) into resealable freezer bags or plastic containers. Drying prevents sticking, and if you use freezer bags, laying the bags on baking sheets before filling them is vital! Put from nine to sixteen in each bag, suck out the excess air, and freeze on the sheet until solid. Store year-round. Thaw persimmons in the refrigerator overnight and eat within 24 hours.

North American

North American persimmons grow wild throughout many states. They are small, about one inch (2.5 cm) in diameter. Treat them as you would a Hachiya. Although tiny, North American persimmons usually contain four or five seeds. Seedless varieties also exist.

Semi-soft

The most common semi-soft variety is the Fuyu. It
has darker flesh than the Hachiya and appears to be a
squashed, square tomato with a crease on each side.
The flesh may contain several seeds and lacks the
sweetness of the Hachiya, but is delicious nevertheless. Fuyus may be eaten while firm but the flavor
improves if you wait. Other semi-soft varieties include the
Yeddo-ichi and Hyakume.

Storing: Semi-soft and firm varieties have the benefit of a lengthy storage
life. They may be refrigerated for up to one month when handled carefully and
set single-layer-high on a flat surface.

Firm

The Zengi is a popular firm variety.

Nutrients: Persimmons are an outstanding source for carotene, vitamin C,
and potassium. They have more vitamin C than oranges, and about one fourth
the carotene of carrots. They are also rich in iron.

Class: Sweet

Physalis

Common Names: Cape gooseberry, Ground cherry,
Pohas, Strawberry tomato

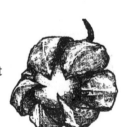

The physalis is a cherry-sized, golden, tomato-like fruit
that comes enveloped in a papery housing. Depending
on the variety, the semi-soft flesh possesses a tangy
to tart flavor. Berry size and husk coloring vary
among the species.

Buying: Select wrapped fruits or those with a full golden hue.
Storing: Store at room temperature.
Class: Acid

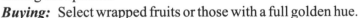

Pineapple *(Ananas comosus)*

The delectable pineapple is a Tropical American native whose appearance and name definitely arouse curiosity in those unfamiliar with the fruit. Spanish explorers coined the name by drawing similarities to the pine cone.[55] Thankfully, pineapples were transplanted to Hawaii where substantial production of the fruit has greatly increased its availability in North America. Hawaii supplies approximately three fourths of world market.

The pineapple holds the distinction of being a perennial herb.[56] Varieties include Sugar Loaf, Red Spanish, and the Smooth Cayenne which is commonly seen in our markets.

Buying/Storing: Hawaiian-grown pineapples generally possess excellent flavor, but those from Costa Rica are superior and have a smaller, tender, edible core. Regardless of the place of origin, obtain a fully ripe fruit.

Green pineapples have pale, acidic flesh, indicating immaturity and poor sugar content. Due to incomplete cellular development, they tend to cut up one's tongue and mouth (jagged cells). The cells of fully ripe fruits become softer, preventing the delicate tissues of the mouth and intestinal tract from being damaged. Sun-ripened fruits are succulent and super-sweet with tender mouth-melting flesh.

🖉 Prematurely harvested pineapples can never attain full potential so it is important to make an educated selection. Choose plump, heavy, firm fruits, with a minimum of thirty percent golden or orange coloring. The sections, "eyes," must be flat and separating from one another. A delightful, fragrant aroma should be emitted without the hint of alcoholic fermentation. Treat pineapples *gently* to prevent bruising and subsequent spoilage. Those that have been subjected to cold temperatures during transport or storage "cut" gray or black.

🖉 To equalize sugar distribution: lay the pineapple on its side and rotate it once or twice a day; or twist off the crown and turn it upside down, giving ample support. Eat when the color improves, or de-crown, wrap in a towel (to prevent cold damage) and refrigerate. Keep for up to three days. For those who desire to eat one half at a time: prepare the lower portion first and leave the top (rind still on) until the next sitting. Place cellophane over the exposed flesh and refrigerate to prevent oxidation and insect problems.

Season: Year-round, peaking from April to July.

Drying: Dry in rings or chunks.

Nutrients: Significant quantities of vitamin C, sulphur, chlorine, and potassium.

📁 Pineapples contain bromalin, a protein-digesting enzyme (proteinase) that aids in the breakdown (metabolism) of proteins. For this very reason, raw nuts and pineapple proves to be an excellent food combination.

Class: Acid

 ☐ *See the recipe section for cutting and serving suggestions!*

Pitanga *(Eugenia uniflora)*

Common Name: Surinam cherry

Pitangas are fragrant, shrub-grown cherries indigenous to South America. The tiny fruits are about one-half the size of a Bing cherry, and narrower, with several distinct ridges. Perfect specimens have glossy, blood-red skins. At this stage a simple touch causes the cherry to release its branch. The tangy flesh is bursting with flavor. An inedible pit occupies the center.

Buying: Unavailable in supermarkets.

Season: Year-round.

Nutrients: Well endowed with vitamin C and carotene. More than double the vitamin C of oranges!

Class: Acid

Pitomba *(Eugenia luschnathiana)*

The rare, delicious pitomba is a Brazilian fruit that grows from a tree-like shrub. The plant thrives in tropical climes and even does well in the Florida Keys. Pitombas appear to be miniature, apricot-colored peaches, about the size of a globe grape and crowned with leaves. The soft, savory flesh brings thoughts of peaches and oranges combined. Treat as you would an apricot.

Buying: Not sold commercially.

Season: May through July.

Class: Sub-acid

Plum *(Prunis salicina, P. domestica)*

Plums are ancient fruits with roots in
Eastern Asia. They decorate small trees
and are adorned with delightful hues of
red, purple, black, yellow, green, or blue.
Their juicy, semi-fibrous flesh can vary with
shades of pink, orange, amber, red, green, or ivory, and
often dually interwoven. Flavors range from tart to sweet.

European plums are small, tart or sweet, and compose the freestone varieties, while Japanese plums attain greater size, are generally sweeter, and fall
into the clingstone category. Small plums are called "prunes" because they
can be dried whole. The dried product is truly the prune.

Buying: Plums bruise easily as evidenced by softness, flesh discoloration,
and fermentation. Select semi-firm fruits without soft spots.

Season: May through early November.

Storing: Ripen at room temperature and keep for up to one month in the
refrigerator.

Drying: Dry "prunes" whole or in halves, and plums in halves or quarters.

Freezing: Wash, halve, and place single-layer-high into freezer bags. Store
for a full year.

Nutrients: A good source for vitamins C, B_2, B_6, and carotene, as well as
potassium.

Class: Sub-acid

❑   *Varieties listed according to the times of availability.*

Black Beaut

A round, medium to large fruit with red, purple, or black skin and juicy,
reddish flesh. Delicately sweet. Look for Black Beauts during May and June.

Santa Rosa

A mid-sized spherical plum with reddish-purple skin and tart-sweet yellow
and red flesh. Available during June and July.

Blackamber

A mid-sized, round fruit with black skin and yellow flesh. Season: June to July.

Laroda

A round, medium plum with crimson skin and succulent, sweet golden flesh.
Marketed in July.

Simka
A medium to large, slightly ovoid fruit with red or purple skin and sweet yellow flesh. July to August availability.

Friar
A large, spherical, purple to black plum with sweet, succulent amber flesh. July through September.

Kelsey
A substantial, heart-shaped green plum that becomes yellow and red upon ripening. The Kelsey has yellowish-green sweet flesh. July to August.

Catilina
A mid-sized, purple plum with a tangy-sweet flavor.

Italian
Familiar to all, these small, ovoid, purple-skinned fruits are called prune plums. Early Italians are available for the first three weeks of August. Late Italians arrive in mid August and last until the third week in September.

Angelino
A medium, slightly pointed, deep red plum with sweet amber flesh. August and September.

Pomegranate *(Punica granatum)*

Pomegranates are ancient shrub-grown fruits native to Asia. A typical fruit is red with similar dimensions to a large apple. Yellow and purple varieties also exist but are rarely seen in North America.

The pomegranate has an uneven and very tough leathery rind that forms a distinct calyx at the bottom. Separating the rind reveals a cluster of sparkling, ruby-red fruits that resemble popcorn kernels. These miniature fruits are tightly packed and divided into sections by thin membranous skins. Each one contains a chewy, edible seed and succulent tangy-sweet juice.

Buying: Select large, heavy, full-colored pomegranates.
Season: Peaks during the winter.
Storing: Stores very well, easily lasting three weeks in the crisper.

Serving: *Method 1* – Slice off the calyx end, score the rind into segments, and then peel each away.

        Method 2 – Simply pull apart.

        Method 3 – Roll on a table or squeeze between your palms until soft. Carefully poke a hole into the rind and suck out the juice.

Nutrients: A good source for potassium.

Class: Acid

Quince *(Cydonia oblonga)*

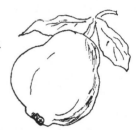

The quince is a firm, bitter fruit, shaped either like a pear or an apple within a pear. The yellow or green skin may have a downy feel. Unfortunately, quinces cannot be enjoyed in the raw state and therefore deserve a recommendation of avoidance.

Class: Acid

Rambutan *(Nephelium lappaceum)*

Rambutan are exotic tree-grown fruits that appear to be from another world. These bizarre, yet strikingly beautiful fruits, are adorned with a number of soft, harmless, deep-red spines. Peeling the skin reveals succulent, translucent flesh whose sweet flavor is reminiscent of the lychee and longan.

Buying: Largest production occurs in Asia.

Storing: Treat as you would lychees.

Nutrients: An excellent source for vitamin C. Notable amounts of potassium and phosphorus.

Class: Sweet

Ramontchi *(Flacourtia indica)*
Common Name: Governor's Plum

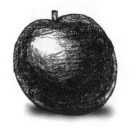

Governor's plums are tree or shrub-grown fruits native to Southern Asia. These walnut-sized, deep purple plums have mild, tender, seeded flesh. Treat as you would a European plum.
Season: Summer
Buying: Not available in supermarkets.
Nutrients: A good source for vitamin C and potassium.
Class: Sub-acid

Sapodilla *(Achras zapota)*
Common Names: Chicozapote, Nispero

The sapodilla or sapota tree is an evergreen indigenous to Mexico and Central America. It has wide-spreading branches and can reach towering heights of 70 feet (21 m). The Florida Keys possesses a suitable growing climate, and those who grow the fruit gather the bounty during the spring and summer; however, this is not a desirable chore considering the size of the tree. Tropical American fruits are harvested throughout the remainder of the year.

🍂 The sapota tree is in itself an agricultural product because it contains a white latex substance called "chicle." Chicle is valued in North America as an ingredient for making chewing gum[57]— thus, the hazardous and undesirable ingredients in chewing gum include refined and artificial sugars, colors and flavors, gelatin and latex. Gum chewing also creates gastrointestinal problems.

Sapodilla fruits are plum to peach-sized with rough brown skins and light or dark tan flesh. When ripe, the flesh is soft, slightly gritty and extremely sweet. A pear blended with brown sugar would closely match the appearance, texture, and outstanding flavor of the flesh. Up to six inedible seeds are situated inside.
Buying: Available in Mexico, Central America, and specialty fruit markets in North America. Select firm fruits and ripen until they yield very easily to gentle pressure.
Storing: When ready, refrigerate for up to two or three days.
Serving: Halve and spoon out the flesh.
Nutrients: A good source for vitamin C and potassium.
Class: Sweet

Soursop *(Annona muricata)*
Common Name: Guanabana

The succulent guanabana is indigenous to Tropical
America. Its relatives include the cherimoya and
sugar apple. Fresh and juiced guanabana is
highly favored in Cuba, Tropical
America, and Miami.

This olive green fruit has the appearance of
a "drooping heart" and grows to a substantial
size, commonly weighing over 5 pounds (2.3
kg) and reaching 1 foot (30 cm) in length. The
teardrop-designed leathery skin is arrayed with a
number of soft, harmless spines.

Buying: Available throughout Tropical
America, and in some specialty fruit markets in the
United States. Select semi-firm, un-punctured fruits
and ripen at room temperature until they yield easily
to gentle pressure. Separation around the stem accompa-
nies softness.

Storing: When ready, they may be refrigerated for up to two days.

Serving: Cut lengthwise from the stem end to expose the fragrant ivory flesh
whose tremendous flavor gives the guanabana the distinction of being one of
the finest fruits.

Nutrients: A good source for vitamin C, niacin, and potassium.

Class: Sub-acid

Star Fruit *(Averrhoa carambola)*
Common Names: Carambola, Five-fingered fruit

The carambola is an exotic tree-grown fruit native to
Malaysia. The prolific tree reaches heights of 20 feet
(6m), and in the summer becomes
adorned with golden, lantern-like
fruits. The fruits have been
perfectly designed so that one can
reach up and pluck them from the
branches using five fingers; hence
the common name—"five-fingered fruit."

Carambolas vary from 4 to 6 inches (10–15 cm) in length and generally contain three to seven elliptic seeds. The edible skin has a decidedly waxy feel, and this adds chewiness to the juicy sub-acid flesh.

Buying: Select golden or deep yellow fruits, free from punctures and signs of decay. Green ones will ripen but with inferior flavor. California, Florida, and Hawaii supply North American demands.

Storing: To prevent cold damage and bruising, wrap ripe carambola in a towel before placing into the crisper. For best flavor, use within two days.

Serving: Make several horizontal slices to create attractive star designs. This brings relevance to the widely-known name—"star fruit."

Drying: Dry as decorative stars.

Freezing: Wash, cut as preferred (removing the seeds), and place into freezer bags; or better yet, simply freeze whole. Use within six months.

Nutrients: An excellent source for carotene. Notable amounts of vitamin C and potassium.

Class: Sub-acid to acid

Sugar Apple *(Annona squamosa)*
Common Names: Sweetsop, Annona

The sugar apple is an outstanding fruit indigenous to Tropical America. As a member of the annonaceous family, its relatives include the cherimoya and soursop. Sugar apples are smaller than these and heart-shaped. The greenish-gray skin is composed of protruding teardrop sections that take on the appearance of armor. This "armor" separates as the fruit ripens, which allows each section to be pulled away to reveal smooth, ivory to white, savory flesh, whose flavor is tremendously sweet.

Season: Summer

Buying: Select semi-firm fruits and ripen at room temperature until they become soft and the skin splits apart. Available in Tropical America, and specialty fruit markets in the United States.

Storing: Keep ripe *annona* in the refrigerator for up to two days.

Nutrients: An excellent source for vitamins C, B_1, B_2, and niacin, as well as calcium and potassium.

Class: Sweet

Tamarillo *(Cyphomandra betacea)*
Common Name: Tree tomato

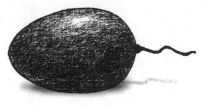

Tamarillos are tomato-like fruits
indigenous to Tropical America.
These oval, apricot-sized tomatoes
have a long stem that appears to be a
tail. When ripe, the bright red or golden
skins yield to pressure. The pulp resem-
bles that of a normal tomato, but is gelatinous and contains flat, lentil-like
black seeds. The flavor is decidedly acidic.
Buying: Avoid bruised, cold-damaged, and poorly colored fruits.
Season: Fall
Storing: Ripen at room temperature before wrapping in a cloth and placing in
the crisper.
Class: Acid

Tamarind *(Tamarindus indica)*

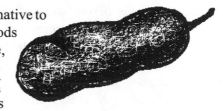

Tamarinds are unusual pod-like fruits native to
Southern Asia. These brown, crispy pods
hang by the thousands from large,
wide-spreading trees, and range from 3
to 6 inches (8–13 cm) in length, and ¾
to 1 inch (1–2.5 cm) in width. The pods
contain sticky, date-like pulp which is
firmly held together by a number of fibers and inedible seeds. Remarkably, the
pulp possesses the highest sugar content of all fruits, while also being the most
acidic. This makes for a tart-sweet flavor comparable to dates drenched in
lemon juice—a combination that brings on a pucker reflex with most people.
    Tamarinds are customarily used for making chutneys, beverages,
preserves, and sauces.
Buying: Sold in a paste or brick, or as fresh pods.
Storing: Keep for months in the refrigerator or freeze for up to eighteen
months.
Nutrients: An outstanding source for potassium. Significant amounts of
thiamine, riboflavin, niacin, iron, calcium, phosphorus, and sodium.
Class: Acid

Vanilla *(Vanilla planifolia)*

The vanilla bean is a vine-grown fruit indigenous to Mexico. The large, flat pods often reach 10 inches (25 cm) in length, and encapsulate black, greasy textured pulp. Once dried, the beans make for a delicious flavoring agent.

☧ Commercially sold extracts contain alcohol (an outright poison), various additives and preservatives, and are very expensive. Untreated dried beans can be obtained in some grocery stores, and in tropical America.
Storing: Freeze, and for best flavor, use within eighteen months.
Class: Sweet

Wampee *(Clausena lansium)*

Wampee are rare, unusual fruits native to Southern China. They grow in clusters (as grapes) on small, v-shaped trees. Yellowish-green skins tightly enclose the translucent, tart-sweet flesh. Treat as you would lychees.
Buying: Not sold in supermarkets.
Class: Sub-acid

Water Apple *(Syzygium aqueum)*

The water apple is a decorative little fruit from India, and can be grown in any subtropical to tropical climate. The fruits develop from a widespread, medium to large tree that bears its bounty during the summer. The bell-shaped, pink fruits average 2 to 3 inches (5–8 cm) in height, and have waxy skins that appear to be melded as one with the flesh (similar to straw-berries). As indicated by the name, water apples are crisp and very juicy—definitely over 90 percent water. The flesh lacks sweetness, but is very satisfying during a heat-wave.
Buying: Not commercially available in this country.
Storing: Place ripe fruits in sealed plastic containers and refrigerate for up to three days.
Class: Sub-acid

White Sapote *(Casimiroa edulis)*
Common Names: Casimiroa, Matasano

The delicious casimiroa grows on a tree common to Mexico. The fruits are spherical and come to a slight point as formed by five shallow creases. They possess Granny Smith apple-coloring when immature, and become off-yellow upon ripening. The smooth, creamy, ivory or orange flesh possesses a flavor reminiscent of an anjou pear. Two to five inedible seeds are situated inside.

Buying: Select semi-firm fruits and ripen at room temperature until they yield to the slightest pressure. Halve and eat with a spoon, or peel the skin and use a fork.

Storing: When ripe, they may be refrigerated for up to two days.

Nutrients: A good source of vitamin C and potassium.

Class: Sub-acid

Dried Fruits

Raisins

·

Dates

·

Figs

·

Prunes

·

Pears

·

Peaches

·

Persimmons

·

Papaya

·

Pineapple

·

Bananas

·

Mango

·

Apples

·

Apricots

·

Cherries

·

Berries

Dried Fruits

Satisfyingly sweet, nutrient dense, and packed with potential energy, dried fruits are valuable additions to a health-minded diet. The nutrients in dried fruits are multiplied three to sixfold over their fresh predecessors, thereby furnishing the requirements (especially calories in the form of sugars) for even the most demanding body, and discouraging unwholesome food cravings. Children, teens, physically fit adults, and those who must endure harsh winters can benefit greatly from these superlative fruits. Sedentary individuals should abstain from generous consumption or suffer the consequences such as gas, bloating, and sugar metabolism problems.

✐ Presoaking dried fruits greatly increases their digestibility. Simply place them in a glass and pour in enough water (preferably distilled) to cover the fruit by one inch. Soak at room temperature or in the refrigerator (prevents bug problems, and bacterial growth in hot weather) until the desired softness is reached. Fresher dates, figs, and raisins may already be soft enough to eat, but it is best to soak or rinse them briefly to remove dirt. Undesirable raisins (those that rotted while drying) are quickly exposed with just a minute or two of presoaking. If your dried fruits have been organically grown and pre-rinsed and sorted, then the soak water will be safe to consume. Drink it as is, or use in shakes, fruit milks, or toppings *(See Recipes)*.

People with sugar metabolism problems (and others as well) may find it beneficial to combine (eat) dried fruits with foods that allow for a more gradual absorption of the fruit sugars. Fresh fruits and thoroughly cooked grains (granola, toast, etc.) combine the best, but lettuce is another possibility since it digests very quickly and replaces some of the water which was evaporated from the fresh fruit (this helps one know when to stop eating). Lettuce is also alkaline-forming and possesses a wide spectrum of nutrients including those that are less abundant in fruits such as vitamin A, calcium, iron, and the B-complex vitamins. An additional benefit of eating lettuce with dried fruits, is that it conveniently cleans the sticky sugars from one's teeth and promotes salivary flow (due to the additional mastication required). The result: healthy teeth and gums, and for some, gentler digestion.

✐ Drinking plenty of water fifteen minutes or more before eating dried fruits (or other concentrated foods) curbs the tendency to overeat, and provides the fluid needed for efficient digestion and free-flowing blood. Taking fluids with one's meal (any foods) is contraindicated because digestive secretions would be diluted, and therefore, could not effectively perform their task. Foods that are not properly digested either ferment or putrefy, and the toxins thus created lay the foundation for disease.

Buying: Every dried fruit, whether in the supermarket or health food store, that does not bear an organically grown label has been made unfit for human consumption. Possible hazards include sulphur, potassium sorbate; fumigants, malathion, and other chemicals; oils, refined sugars, bleaches, and pasteurization. Avoid these hazards and save money by purchasing bulk quantities of organically grown dried fruits from a natural food distributor. Organically grown raisins are very inexpensive when bought in quantities of 25 or 30 pounds (11.3 or 13.6 kg), and pound for pound, are about one-third the cost of pre-bagged raisins sold in supermarkets. To locate a natural food distributor who meets your needs, search the telephone directory or find out who supplies the health food stores in your area.

▱ Be watchful: some organically grown dried fruits (and all dried fruits sold as bulk in the supermarkets) have been oiled. Oil (any fat) taken with dried fruit (any sugar) could be a lethal combination for some because it causes blood levels of cholesterol and triglycerides to remain high for extended periods of time.[58, 59] The blood becomes thick, fatty, and sluggish, which encourages atherosclerosis, clotting, and cellular death. Excessive consumption of oils (not just saturated animal fats) can cause obesity, heart and circulatory diseases, and even cancer—carcinogens form when oils are subjected to high temperatures.

☠ The pesticides used on non-organically grown fresh fruits are never washed off before drying, and they become concentrated during the dehydration process. It has been common practice to dry grapes (and most assuredly other fruits) on malathion-treated trays in an attempt to prevent insect problems—pesticides are ineffective, as was shown in *Pesticides* in Part 1. The grapes (or other fresh fruits) absorb the malathion, and the tainted finished product, "raisins," are sold to an unsuspecting public.

What about sulphur?

Sulphite compounds (six common ones are used including sulphur dioxide) are applied to improve the feel and appearance of foods, in order to increase sales and profits. Sulphur enables dried fruits to be packaged with a higher water content—you pay for the water.[60]

Sulphur dioxide and its salts have toxic, mutagenic, and anti-nutritional effects.[61] One study by the United States Department of Agriculture proved that sulphur dioxide causes kidney problems, destroys red and white blood cells, leaches calcium and other minerals from the body, inflames the mucous membranes of the mouth and intestinal tract, and increases uric acid levels. Other symptoms included nausea, albumenuria, sensation of cold, headache, backache, belching, malaise, anemia, listlessness, and dull eyes.[62] Anaphylactic shock, abdominal pain, dizziness, and hives are other serious symptoms.[63] Many deaths have been reported due to the ingestion of foods preserved with sulphite-based compounds—27 to the FDA in about a one year period,[64] and undoubtedly, many others occurred where sulphite poisoning went unsuspected.

One anti-nutritional effect of sulphites is that they cause negative interactions with a number of vitamins (especially thiamine and folic acid).[65] This explains why sulphite compounds cannot be legally used in North America on most fresh fruits and vegetables (just since 1986); however, grapes and potatoes are exceptions. Excluding grapes and potatoes from this law is perplexing since they are both above-average sources of thiamine. Dried fruits can be (and most are) legally treated with sulphur even though most people eat them raw. Disturbing, considering the fact that the thiamine and other nutrients are multiplied three to sixfold in dried fruits. The result, even greater losses.

Shredded coconut and nuts can also be treated with sulphur. All other foods (processed ones including animal products) contain the greatest amounts of sulphites. For example, most hamburgers analyzed from restaurants were found to have sulphites, some at elevated levels.[66] Obviously, junk foods should be avoided at all costs.

A second anti-nutritional effect of sulphites, namely toxic by-product formation, occurs when high-fat foods are sulphured before storage.[67] Dried fruits that have been oiled could be subject to this effect.

To magnify the senselessness of sulphite and other preservative treatments given to dried fruits, one need only consider that dried fruits are not vulnerable to rapid spoilage because they have low moisture contents. Whenever necessary, refrigeration can be used to greatly increase their storage life.

Space prevents further discussion of the other harmful treatments applied to dried fruits.

❏   Since organically grown dried fruits are reasonably priced (when bought in bulk quantities), one who purchases them not only invests in their own health, but literally in the health of mankind because pesticides poison our waters, soils, air, and foods.

Serving: All non-organically grown dried fruits should be washed thoroughly before consumption. Organic fruits are best rinsed or soaked briefly.
Storing: For optimal quality, extended storage life, and the avoidance of insect problems, keep short-term needs in the refrigerator and freeze all other supplies. "Frozen" dried fruits are best used within eighteen months but will keep longer if necessary. Dried fruits do not actually freeze due to their low water contents, and therefore, can be warmed very quickly.

✍ Dried fruits become "sugared" when subjected to warmer temperatures and humidity variances. Sugaring is evident when a white coating or crystals have formed on the exterior. These natural sugars do not indicate spoilage; in fact, the fruit becomes sweeter.

Class: Sweet

Raisins (Vitis vinifera, V. labrusca)

Raisins have been used as a significant food source since 1000 years before the birth of Jesus.[68] Spanish explorers brought grapes to California in the 1700's, but they were not dried into raisins until 1873 when a heat wave dried most of the grape crop on the vines. Thus, raisins were "rediscovered."[69]

It takes approximately 4½ pounds of fresh grapes to produce one pound of raisins;[70] therefore, raisins are an economical food choice. Raisins have remarkable keeping qualities with incredible resistance to molds, bacteria, and pathogenic organisms, and possess the ability to remain soft for extended periods of time. Raisins are well endowed with natural sugars—low in sucrose and high in fructose. Their water content is minimal at 15 to 18 percent.[71]

Serving: Be sure to thoroughly wash all non-organically grown raisins—see the previous information on presoaking.

Nutrients: Raisins are an outstanding source for iron, potassium, and calcium.

□ *Raisins that have been produced from seeded grapes are to be sought after because the original grape stock may not have been tampered with through the centuries. The seeded, tangy flavored Muscat was grown at least as far back as 1000 B.C.,[72] and therefore, it could be one of the only original grapes left in the world. The Muscat accounted for most of the Californian grape crop until the introduction of the Thompson seedless grape in 1876.[73] Unfortunately, the Muscat raisin has all but disappeared from the North American marketplace, thus leaving the organic Thompson as the best alternative in most locales. Further research is required to find out whether the Thompson or any other seedless varieties have been developed without crossing two varieties together. Unless organically grown, seedless varieties will contain pesticide residues and other chemicals.*

Muscat

Generally sun-dried and preservative-free. Mechanically removed *seeds.* Muscats possess a distinctive tangy-sweet flavor. The Muscat and the Lexia are the two best raisins because they are produced from seeded grapes and possess outstanding flavors.

Lexia
Sun-dried, preservative-free, *seeded* raisins. Superb flavor with unmatched sweetness! Regrettably, poor crops and the unfortunate switch to more seedless varieties has greatly limited or nullified marketing in North America.

Sun-dried, Natural Seedless
Thompson Seedless. Packaged product is generally, but not always, un-oiled. Thompsons that are sold in the bulk food sections of supermarkets have been unnecessarily oiled and sulphured, and may contain potassium sorbate. Organically grown Thompsons are available at reasonable prices, especially when bought in bulk quantities; however, it could be a hybrid. Smaller prepackaged bags and boxes of organically grown Thompson raisins are sold in some supermarkets.

Golden Seedless
Beware: Air-dried Thompson grapes that have been laced with sulphur dioxide to create that eye-catching, golden color. They are generally preserved in potassium sorbate, and could be oiled.

Dipped Seedless
Thompson Seedless that were nutritionally sacrificed in a hot water soup before air-drying. Potassium sorbate and oil may have been applied.

Monukka
Dark, richly sweet, and very soft when fresh. Organically grown sun-dried Monukkas can be ordered from a number of specialty distributors.

Red Flame
Sun-dried flame grapes. Outstanding tangy-sweet flavor. Organically grown product is available but it is difficult to find an oil-free source.

Sultana
Sultanas are generally sun-dried, but could be covered in oil and potassium sorbate. Less sweet. Produced from a seedless grape—the first of its kind.[74]

Figs, Dates, and Apricots are listed under their own headings, and ***Prunes*** are discussed under ***Plums***. Other commonly available dried fruits include apples, pineapple, papaya, peaches, pears, persimmons, bananas, cherries, cranberries, blueberries, and mangos.

❑   *Drying your own fruits allows for even greater variety.*

Nuts and Seeds

❖

Almond

•

Brazil

•

Cashew

•

Chestnut

•

Filberts and Hazelnuts

•

Macadamia

•

Peanut

•

Pecan

•

Pine Nut

•

Pistachio

•

Walnut

•

Pumpkin Seeds

•

Sesame Seeds

•

Sunflower Seeds

Nuts and Seeds

Nuts are delicious, satisfying foods that probably date back to the beginning of time. Earliest Biblical evidence occurs in Genesis 43:11, where "nuts and almonds" are mentioned [pistachios (margin) and almonds]. Many varieties exist, and offer a wide diversity of tastes.

Nuts have been placed in the same botanical class as fruits; however, "nut-fruits" deserve a separate classification because the edible portions are the seeds themselves. Nuts, being perfectly designed foods, have sealed, hard shell encasements that protect them from pests and bacteria, environmental conditions, and the chemicals sprayed by unconcerned growers. Besides ensuring growth and sterility, the shells lock out oxygen, and this helps greatly in preserving freshness. Up until mechanical shelling, the extra work of cracking nuts helped to prevent overeating. A solid reason to purchase in-shell nuts.

Being highly concentrated, nuts and seeds supply an abundance of vitamins, minerals, and fiber, and are an unbeatable source for proteins and unsaturated fats (fatty acids: linoleic, linolenic, oleic, arachidonic, etc.). Moderate consumption enables the body to make use of these riches. Nuts and seeds are easily digested when chewed thoroughly—to a smooth, creamy chyme. Those who cannot chew nuts and seeds to this point should eat them as butters. Under normal circumstances, when nuts are eaten in proper quantity and thoroughly chewed, they will not putrefy in the digestive tract—unlike flesh foods which not only putrefy and contain urea and uric acid, but also cause abnormal bacteria to proliferate (forms that lead to cancer). However, overeating on nuts is a sin (as is overeating on any food) that results in the formation of toxins, which in turn poison the blood and cause disease. Since nuts are high in protein and fat, the effects of overeating will be manifest quickly and markedly: headache, vertigo (dizziness), unclear thinking, malaise (uneasiness), and exhaustion.

Evidently, due to their dense nutrient nature, nuts must be eaten in very small amounts; not as snacks, but rather with other foods to form satisfying meals (see *Food Combining*). The ideal quantity per day depends on one's weight, activity level, age, and the other high protein and fat foods contained in the diet. The weather conditions also play a role since more calories are required during colder weather. Children and physical laborers can use more. One-eighth to three ounces per day represents a broad range. Putting to practice the information given thus far will do one little good unless nuts and seeds are eaten as provided in nature—raw. Cooking makes nuts partially or wholly indigestible and destroys or deranges the nutrients.

🗀 Nuts are excellent nerve, brain, and bone-building foods. Their high quality fats provide lubrication for the joints, and structure and flexibility to literally every cell. Carefully note that nuts and seeds are cholesterol-free.

Studies have found nuts to protect against fatal and non-fatal coronary heart disease. A study on one population group found that those who consumed nuts most frequently (five or more times per week in moderate amounts) had 53 percent less risk of dying from coronary heart disease.[75] Not surprisingly, whole raw nuts appear to have the greatest impact.[76] *Note that nuts and seeds should take the place of flesh, eggs, and dairy products.*

☠ Dry roasted and other processed peanuts or nuts may contain MSG, BHA, mono and diglycerides, modified food starch, and salt. The suspected health hazards from these substances include cancer, birth defects, liver diseases, genetic mutations, and lung damage.[77]

Buying: Stock up on in-shell and shelled nuts during the fall and winter. Buy from a natural food distributor, health food store, or the supermarket.

Bulk food sections in most supermarkets carry raw, unsalted, oil-free nuts and seeds. Wash or soak these to remove dirt and possible pesticide residues. Unshelled nuts are by far the safest, but time and the availability of certain varieties may factor into your choices.

Storing: Place nuts and seeds into glass jars or resealable freezer bags and store them in the freezer. They do not actually freeze due to their low water content. Assuming that you purchased fresh product, in-shell nuts may be stored in the freezer for up to $1\frac{1}{2}$ years, and shelled ones for up to ten months. Those kept at room temperature (particularly shelled ones) quickly become stale and rancid, and can develop free radicals or carcinogenic molds (see *Peanuts* for aflatoxins and advice).

Class: Protein (unless specified as starch)

Almond (Prunus amygdalus)

The almond is a delicately flavored, elliptic nut whose kernel comes loosely packaged in a pitted shell.

Nutrients: Almonds exceed all other nuts for calcium, and are one of the highest sources known to man, having double the calcium of cow's milk, and in a state that is condu- cive to human health. The calcium in cow's milk is largely unavailable.[78]

Next to kelp, almonds top the list for magnesium, and are an outstanding source for potassium, iron, phosphorus, niacin, and riboflavin. Almonds contain 19.5 g of protein and 54.2 g of fat per 100 g portion.

Almonds, coconuts, and chestnuts are the only nuts that leave an alkaline ash upon metabolism, and of these, the almond possesses the highest alkalinity. Almonds also digest quicker than all other nuts.

Brazil Nut *(Bertholletia exselsa)*

The Brazil is an oily, richly flavored nut whose ivory meat (edible portion) is encased in a hard, wedge-shaped, burnt-brown shell. The shells are difficult to crack and leave a russet stain on one's fingers. The tight skin that surrounds the meat may be scraped off if so desired.

Buying: Avoid shelled nuts that have dark or burnt areas because this indicates spoilage. Brazils are highly perishable so buy a small sample first to check for rancidity.

Nutrients: Brazils are higher in fat and lower in protein than most nuts—a desirable composition due to the high quality of nut fats, and the fact that most people get far more protein than required.

Brazils are an excellent source for calcium, potassium, magnesium, phosphorus, sulphur, and B-complex vitamins.

Cashew *(Anacardium occidentale)*

Cashew "meats" are semi-crunchy and have a delicious, slightly sweet flavor which rates second only to the macadamia nut. They can attain incredible lengths of 3 inches (7.6 cm), although those commercially available are usually one-third this size. Interestingly, the nut hangs below the "cashew apple," an edible, apple or pear-shaped fleshy portion. A poisonous husk surrounds the nut. Before the husk is removed it must be heated to neutralize the cardol and anacardic acids.[79]

☞ Cashews are related to poison ivy but do not let that stop you from partaking.

Buying: Avoid tiny, shriveled nuts because they are flavorless and probably old.

Nutrients: The quick heating process applied to remove the husks does not have a marked effect on the meat inside, and therefore, raw cashews are an excellent food. Cashews contain generous amounts of iron, potassium, magnesium, phosphorus, and B-complex vitamins.

Chestnut *(Castanea dentata)*

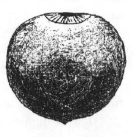

Chestnuts have a different chemical composition than other nuts and should be classed separately. They are extremely starchy, and contain just 1.5 g of fat and 2.9 g of protein per 100 g portion. Put into perspective, this is one-fiftieth the fat and one-sixth the protein of the almond. Chestnuts require light boiling or roasting to improve digestibility.
Nutrients: An excellent source for potassium and B-complex vitamins. Chestnuts are alkaline in metabolic reaction.
Class: Starch

Coconut *(see **Coconut** in the Fruit Guide)*

Filberts and Hazelnuts *(Corylus)*

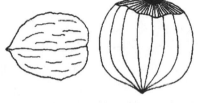

The filbert is a brown to dark russet nut with a flattened crown and stout body. Its hard shell provides a roomy shelter for the tasty meat. The tight skin may be scraped off if so desired. Hazelnuts generally have smaller dimensions than filberts, and are therefore sold pre-shelled.
Buying: Buy in-shell filberts during the fall and winter.
Nutrients: Relatively high in fat and lower in protein—an excellent ratio (see *Brazil Nut* for explanation). Filberts are an exceptional source for calcium, and are rich in potassium, iron, phosphorus, magnesium, sulphur, and B-complex vitamins.

Macadamia *(Macadamia ternifolia)*

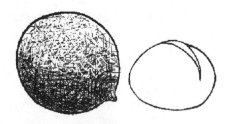

Few will disagree that macadamias are the finest nuts given to man. Not surprisingly, the tastiest nut also possesses the hardest shell, requiring a heavy-duty nutcracker to get at the meat inside. Most people prefer to buy pre-shelled nuts. The delectable ivory meats are oily with a semi-crunchy consistency.

Macadamias were first grown in Australia before being transplanted to Hawaii. California produces a small crop.

Buying: Macadamias are most reasonably priced in South Africa, Australia, and Hawaii. For lower prices, combine your purchasing power with others and buy in bulk.

Nutrients: As far as nuts go, macadamias contain the least amount of protein, and are rich in high-quality fatty acids, phosphorus, potassium, iron, and B-complex vitamins.

Peanut *(Arachis hypogaea)*
Common Names: Goober, Groundpea, Groundnut

Contrary to popular belief, peanuts are not nuts, but legumes; nevertheless, we will discuss them here due to their popularity and mistaken identity. Peanuts grow underground while true nuts grow on trees.

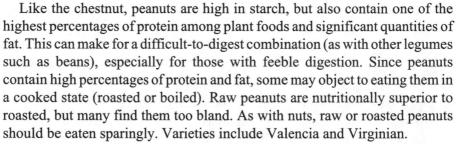

Like the chestnut, peanuts are high in starch, but also contain one of the highest percentages of protein among plant foods and significant quantities of fat. This can make for a difficult-to-digest combination (as with other legumes such as beans), especially for those with feeble digestion. Since peanuts contain high percentages of protein and fat, some may object to eating them in a cooked state (roasted or boiled). Raw peanuts are nutritionally superior to roasted, but many find them too bland. As with nuts, raw or roasted peanuts should be eaten sparingly. Varieties include Valencia and Virginian.

☠ Incorrectly stored peanuts (and many other foods) can develop carcinogenic molds called aflatoxins—moldy animal feeds (peanut meal, grains, soy, etc.) are a major problem that results in contaminated animal products. Studies show a significant increase in liver cancers among those who consume diets high in aflatoxins.[80] To prevent alflatoxin formation, growers, packers, and consumers alike must store peanuts (and other susceptible foods) in a cool, low-moisture environment. Unfortunately, many countries (especially tropical ones) do not take adequate precautions, and this results in peanuts (foods) with high levels of aflatoxins. The United States and Canada have much higher standards than most countries, and therefore, domestic peanuts afford little risk. In past years, Canadian-grown peanuts have tested aflatoxin-free.[81] Unless you are sure of the source, avoid all peanuts that have not been produced in North America. *Always* discard moldy, discolored, shriveled, or damaged peanuts (and nuts) because they contain the highest levels of aflatoxins. Sort through peanuts and nuts soon after they are purchased and store them in the refrigerator or freezer.

Storing: Refrigerate or freeze peanuts, removing desired portions as the need arises.

Nutrients: Raw peanuts are the highest whole food source for niacin.

Class: Starch

Pecan (Carya illinoinensis)

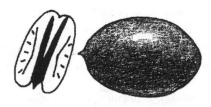

The pecan is a delectable nut with a chewy texture and rich flavor. A brown edible skin tightly envelopes the irregular shaped meat.

Buying: Smaller varieties possess superior flavor.

Nutrients: Possesses a low protein, high fatty acid ratio. Significant amounts of potassium, phosphorus, magnesium, iron, calcium, B-complex vitamins, and carotene.

Pine Nut–Pinon–Pignolia (Pinus species)

Pignolias are the seeds from certain types of pine cones. The tiny tooth-shaped meats are tender and full-flavored, but generally too expensive to justify a purchase.

Nutrients: Very concentrated, only second to the soybean in protein as far as plant foods are concerned. Pignolias also contain an abundance of B-complex vitamins, calcium, magnesium, phosphorus, and iron.

Pistachio (Pistacia vera)

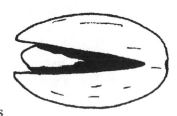

The pistachio has a rich, striking flavor that gives it the distinction of being one of the finest of nuts. The outer shells are naturally ivory, smooth, almond-shaped, and generally split open to expose the attractive green meats and brown skins. Pistachios are native to the Middle East. California produces a substantial crop.

☠ Avoid pistachios that have been died red. Red Dye 40 (Allura Red AC) is suspected of causing cancer and birth defects.[82]

Nutrients: Pistachios are rich in iron and potassium, and contain significant quantities of phosphorus, calcium, magnesium, and the B-complex vitamins.

Walnut (Juglans regia-English, J. nigra-Black)

Walnuts are oily and possess a flavor similar to that of the pecan, although less pronounced.
Buying: English walnuts are superior to the Black varieties which are generally sold pre-shelled.
Nutrients: Walnuts are a tremendous source for B-complex vitamins and linolenic acid (the most beneficial fatty acid), and contain generous supplies of potassium, magnesium, iron, and phosphorus.

Pumpkin Seeds (Cucurbita)

Pumpkin seeds have a distinct, heavy flavor that is either enjoyed or disliked altogether.
Buying: Purchase from a health food store or dry your own.
Nutrients: Extremely high in protein—only surpassed by the pine nut. With the exception of seaweed, pumpkin seeds contain more phosphorus than all other raw, whole foods! They are also an excellent source for B-complex vitamins.

Sesame Seeds (Sesamum indicumor, S. orientale)

Sesame seeds are chewy, herb-produced, miniature white or black seeds. You may have eaten these wonderfully flavored seeds as a ground paste called tahini.

Buying: Purchase raw, hulled seeds and use them with fruits, grains, or select vegetables. Ground seeds are called tahini. Sesame seeds are inexpensive.

Nutrients: Raw sesame seeds are the highest known source of organic calcium on this earth! They have ten times the amount found in cow's milk! Sesame seeds are also an outstanding source for iron, B-complex vitamins, potassium, and phosphorus, and contain notable amounts of magnesium.

Sunflower Seeds *(Helianthus annuus)*

Hardly needing description, sunflower seeds are minuscule, gray to silvery seeds with a rich, delectable flavor. Use them with fruits, grains, or select vegetables.

Buying: Purchase raw, in-shell or hulled seeds. Very inexpensive.

Nutrients: Sunflower seeds are the best raw, whole food source of thiamine—the good disposition vitamin—and are rich in potassium, iron, phosphorus, silicon, calcium, and all other B vitamins.

Vegetable Fruits

❖

Cucumber

·

Eggplant

·

Sweet Pepper

·

Summer Squash

·

Tomato

Fruits or Vegetables?

What are the distinguishing characteristics that determine whether a food should be classified as a fruit or a vegetable? From one point of view, if a food is the product of a tree or plant and contains seeds within itself, then it is a fruit. With this definition in mind, one could reason that cucumbers, eggplant, peppers, squash, and tomatoes are fruits, and could be combined as such. On-the-other-hand, natural inclination would indicate that these foods (except tomatoes perhaps) are vegetables since one would not normally eat them with fruits. Undoubtedly, tomatoes, due to their consistency and rapid digestion time, can easily be classed and combined as a fruit. Nevertheless, for the benefit of the reader, each of these foods will be discussed.

Buying: As always, strive to grow at least some of your own produce. Vegetable-fruits grow well in cooler climates where fruit trees are unsuccessful, so everyone can grow something—even in a pot, planter, or bucket on a balcony.

☠ To increase eye-appeal, most of the vegetable-fruits sold in supermarkets are heavily waxed or oiled. The waxes contain fungicides and lock in all the chemicals and dirt that lie on the fruit's surface. *Never* eat skins that have been waxed (see *Pesticides* in Part 1), and wash oils off with warm water and produce soap. Buy from farmer's markets where organically grown produce is often available, or at the very least, that which is unwaxed.

Storing: To retain freshness and greatly extend storage life, place all vegetable-fruits (except tomatoes) in tightly sealed, plastic containers and refrigerate. Use them quickly—within five days.

Drying: Simply dry into crispy chips or rings. These not only have outstanding flavor but are free from oil, salt, additives, and preservatives. Dried vegetable-fruits contain generous quantities of vitamins and minerals.

Cucumber *(Cucumis sativus)*

Cucumbers are ancient fruits which belong to the same family as watermelons. Today, we have numerous varieties with differing characteristics. They can be finger-sized or up to two feet long. The skins may be green, yellow, or even white, with a smooth, ridged, or warty feel. The mildly sweet or bland flesh can vary in consistency from meaty to seedy.

Buying: Select firm cucumbers!

Nutrients: Outstanding sources for silicon, bromine, sulphur, and chlorine.

Class: Neutral

Slicing

Slicing cucumbers are plump, usually dark green, and full of seeds. Beware: supermarket product is always heavily waxed.

Pickling

Pickling cucumbers are tiny, green, and warty, with crispy, dense flesh. They are superbly flavored and may not be waxed if obtained from a local source.

Long-English

Long-English cucumbers are green, ridged, and elongated, with a bland to semi-sweet flavor. They could be waxed but the skins are quite thin and can be easily peeled, (thus substantially reducing one's pesticide intake).

Eggplant (Solanum melongena)

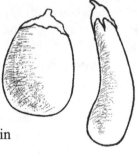

The common eggplant is oblong and bulbous with a dark purple hue. Its spongy white flesh is semisweet or bland, and riddled with tiny, disklike, edible seeds. Contrary to popular belief, eggplants can be enjoyed raw (when tender), and this affords the opportunity to obtain the full complement of nutrients.

Japanese eggplants are light to deep purple, and elongated, often reaching a foot in length. They are exceptionally flavored and great for out-of-hand eating, especially as raw *Eggplant Roll-ups* (see recipes).

✎ Eggplant oxidizes *very* quickly: Thick varieties should be sliced immediately before serving (or preparation), while Japanese eggplants may be sliced during one's meal. Avoid leftovers.

Buying: With either type select soft, spongy fruits, free from decay, discoloration, brown spots, and skin breaks. Minor wrinkling is inconsequential.

Nutrients: Eggplants are rich in chlorine, sulphur, and potassium.

Class: Neutral

Sweet Pepper *(Capsicum frutescens)*

Sweet peppers are hollow fruits of differing bulbous
configurations. As many as six pronounced formations create visual appearances ranging from trian-
gular to hexagonal. Skin colors include green,
yellow, red orange, white, brown, and purple. Fresh
peppers have firm, crisp, juicy flesh.

Use sweet peppers to add flavor to a dressing or
recipe.

Buying: Select firm, deeply-colored fruits, free from
cracks and signs of decay. Green peppers are generally the least expensive to
buy but red ones are often reasonably priced as well. All other sweet peppers
are generally too expensive to justify a purchase.

☠ Test results consistently show peppers to have the highest pesticide levels
amongst produce, with imports being by far the worst. Most of these chemicals are systemic, meaning that they are actually in the flesh itself. To be wise,
grow your own peppers (easily done), visit farmer's markets (ask questions),
and limit your intake of supermarket peppers, *especially imports*. Wash
store-bought peppers thoroughly.

Nutrients: Green peppers are an excellent source for vitamin C, having more
than $2\frac{1}{2}$ times that of an orange! They also contain notable amounts of
carotene and potassium.

Red peppers are an outstanding source for vitamin C and carotene, having
four times the vitamin C of an orange and almost half the carotene of a carrot!
Class: Sub-acid

Squash *(Cucurbita pepo)*

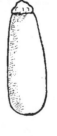
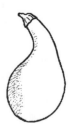

Young summer squash are tender and delicious
in the raw state. Crooknecks have deep yellow
skin and a curved neck, while zucchinis are dark
green and of varying forms. Each has its own
semi-crunchy, delicately flavored flesh.

Buying: Pick small, colorful fruits free from
decay.

Nutrients: Good sources for carotene, potassium, and
niacin.

Class: Neutral

Tomato *(Lycopersicon esculentum)*

Although low in sugar, tomatoes can burst with flavor. Vine-ripened tomatoes are unsurpassed. If you cannot remember the last time you bit into a meaty, tangy-sweet tomato—then it is time to start gardening. Tomatoes must be vine-ripened and garden-grown to achieve full potential. Whenever possible, grow your own. Even if you do not have a garden, tomatoes (and practically anything else) can easily be grown in buckets. Buy from farmer's markets in all other cases. There are four basic types of tomatoes, and from smallest to largest they are: cherry, plum, medium, and beefsteak.

🖊 Home-growers should locate a seed supplier who carries heirloom varieties. Brandywine tomatoes are mammoth heirloom fruits that have an incredible tangy-sweet flavor.

Buying: Today's *manufactured* supermarket tomatoes *generally* deserve a recommendation of avoidance because they are flavorless, covered in pesticides, and decay overnight—look for local product. Hot house tomatoes also lack flavor, but choose them over field varieties because they contain fewer pesticides and have predictable ripening and storage qualities. Cherry and plum (Roma etc.) tomatoes that have not been picked too early may be worth purchasing.

☠ See *Genetic Engineering* in Part 1 for tomato cautions.

Tomatillos are small, green, tomato-like fruits that are surrounded by a papery housing (comparable to the *Physalis* illustration). They have a powerful tangy-tart flavor and are excellent in salsas and dressings. Unlike tomatoes, tomatillos can be kept for weeks in the refrigerator.

Storing: Tomatoes are cold sensitive and should not be refrigerated. Ripen them at 60–65°F (16-18°C) with a relative humidity around 90 percent. For best results, keep ripe fruits at 55–60°F (13-16°C).

Nutrients: Ripe tomatoes surpass all whole raw foods for organic chlorine, and contain significant levels of carotene, vitamin C, bromine, sulphur, potassium, and silicon.

Class: Acid

Part 3

The
Recipe
Guide

Recipes

❖

Shakes • Fruit Pops • Banana Pops • Fruit Puddings,

Soups and Sauces • Jams • Toppings • Fruit Medleys

Ice Creams • Ice Cream Parfait • Super Banana Split

Candy • Fudge • Banana Logs • Cookies • Pies

Papaya Boats • Nut, Seed, and Fruit Milks • Nut or

Seed Butters • Nut, Seed, or Peanut Plums • Melon Boats

"Porcupine" Mango • Cutting and Serving Pineapple

Salad Dressings • Salsas, Dips, and Guacamole

Stuffed Peppers and Tomatoes • Eggplant Roll-ups

Creamy Seven Soup

Introduction

The following recipes consist entirely of raw, natural, plant foods (barring optional ingredients), and each is free from cholesterol, refined sugars, additives, preservatives, irritants, and every other harmful substance associated with the food processing industry. One must use fresh, raw ingredients or the above statement does not apply. The recipes serve as a guide and provide many options, encouraging you to experiment and to create nutritious, eye-appealing alternatives to match your own tastes. Use raw food recipes as a steppingstone in your quest for the optimal diet—one abundantly supplied with unprocessed fresh fruits, vegetables, and moderate amounts of raw nuts and seeds. By adhering to a temperate diet based on raw fruits, your body will naturally reward you with weight loss (or normalization) and maintenance, additional energy, and high-level mental acuity. Therefore, the following recipes will prove valuable as you *begin* transforming the way you eat, feel, look, and think!

Be aware that frozen, cooked, or fragmented foods (juiced, blended, shredded, processed) are compromises to the ideal (whole raw foods) and therefore should not constitute a large portion of one's diet. Home-processed natural foods can be valuable additions, but the emphasis should be placed on whole, room-temperature fruits (foods).

The ice creams, cold shakes (if you decide to make them cold), and any other cold-prepared foods described below should be *eaten slowly* so that they may be warmed and thoroughly mixed with saliva before being swallowed. Cold foods must be warmed before digestion can effectively proceed. Do your best to minimize cold foods.

Also note that a number of the recipes give the option of combining sweet fruits with nuts (including coconut) or seeds. This difficult-to-digest combination will prove troublesome for some. Refer to *Food Combining* for an explanation.

☠ Before creating any of these delicious recipes, see the section on water in Part 1. Also refer to *Buying and Eating Fruits for Nourishment* for information on juices, and *Obtaining Safe Foods* for instruction in reducing your intake of pesticides.

Shakes

fresh, frozen, or dried fruits
distilled water or fruit juice
raw nuts or seeds (optional)

The following shakes are nutrient dense and quick to prepare. Those based on sub-acid fruits and melons are light and refreshing, while the sweet ones are satisfying and supply long-lasting energy. The volume of water that you use depends on the size of the shake(s) and the desired consistency. For ease of digestion, room temperature shakes are recommended. If a cool shake is preferred on a hot day, you can use cold water and room temperature fruit; warm water, ice cubes, and fruit; or warm water and frozen fruit. Fresh-squeezed juices may also be used. Simply blend 1½ cups (355 ml) of water (or juice) with a few bananas (or other fruits) and then add extra fruit, flavorings, water, or ice cubes until you have developed the perfect shake. Shakes made with juicier fruits need little if any water.

Use bananas as a base for thick, sweet shakes. Shakes that contain dried fruits or firm dates require some preplanning: Soak these fruits in a glass of distilled water until they are soft enough to allow for easy blending, thus preventing the appliance from being overworked. Dried fruits may be soaked at room temperature, or in the refrigerator if you have insect problems. Use the *sweet soak water* (if the fruit was clean and untreated) as part of the shakes water requirements.

Shakes should be considered as meals and not drinks, and are therefore best taken slowly, and apart from vegetables, legumes, and animal products (see *Food Combining* in Part 1).

The author does not recommend liquid diets (especially commercially prepared liquid protein diets); however, those with dental problems can generally use shakes to great advantage.

Sweet Shakes

Banana — Date
(2–5 bananas; 6—14 pitted, presoaked, or fresh dates; distilled water to reach desired consistency)

Banana — Raisin
(2–5 bananas, presoaked raisins to taste, distilled water)

Banana — Fig
(2–5 bananas, fresh or soaked-till-soft dried figs, distilled water. Be sure to remove the stems from the figs before blending)

Banana — Mango
(2–5 bananas, 1 ripe mango, distilled water as needed)

Banana — Carob
(3–5 bananas, 2–4 heaping tablespoons of raw sugar-free carob powder, distilled water to taste)

Banana — Blueberry (or other berry)
(3–5 bananas, 1–2 cups (237–473 ml) of berries, distilled water to preferred consistency)

Banana — Pear
(3–4 bananas, 2–3 pears, distilled water to desired consistency)

Banana — Papaya
(3–4 bananas, 1 papaya, and just enough distilled water to make creamy)

Banana — Persimmon
(3–4 bananas; 2–4 super-ripe, de-stemmed persimmons; and just enough distilled water to allow for easy blending)

Banana — Pineapple
(2–4 bananas, ½–1 fresh pineapple or the juice from the Skinless Alligator method of "Cutting and Serving Pineapple" as described later in the recipe section, distilled water if needed)

Banana — Stone Fruit
(3–5 bananas; 2–4 peaches, nectarines, apricots, or plums; distilled water to desired consistency)

Banana — Vanilla
(3–5 bananas, untreated vanilla bean—ground or minced, and distilled water to preferred consistency)

Sub-Acid Shakes

❑   *Use any type of citrus fruit in place of oranges.*

Orange — Berry
(4–7 de-seeded oranges or 6–12 ounces of fresh-squeezed juice, ½–1½ cups (118–355 ml) of preferred berries, distilled water if needed)

Orange — Pineapple
(2–4 de-seeded oranges or fresh-squeezed juice, ½–1 fresh pineapple or the juice from the Skinless Alligator method of "Cutting and Serving Pineapple" as described later in the recipe section)

Orange — Stone Fruit
(3–6 de-seeded oranges or preferred quantity of freshly squeezed orange juice, 2–4 pieces of your favorite stone fruits)

Orange — Pineapple—Kiwi
(2–3 de-seeded oranges, 1–2 kiwis, ½ of a fresh pineapple or the juice from the Skinless Alligator method of "Cutting and Serving Pineapple" as described in the recipe section, fresh-squeezed juice if desired)

Papaya — Orange
(1 large or 2 small, seeded papayas, 3–6 de-seeded oranges, distilled water or fresh-squeezed juice to desired consistency)

Papaya — Stone Fruit
1 large or 2 small papayas; 2–4 peaches, nectarines, apricots, or plums; distilled water or fresh-squeezed juice to preferred consistency)

Papaya — Mango
(1 large or 2 small papayas, 1–2 fully ripe mangos, just enough distilled water or fresh-squeezed juice to make it creamy)

Strawberry — Stone Fruit
(1–2 cups (237–473 ml) of strawberries; 2–4 peaches, nectarines, apricots, or plums; freshly squeezed juice of preference or distilled water)

Mango — Berry
(1–2 cups (237–473 ml) of berries, 1–3 mangos, and freshly squeezed juice of preference or distilled water)

Pineapple — Pear
(½ of a fresh pineapple or the juice from the Skinless Alligator method of "Cutting and Serving Pineapple" as described later in the recipe section, 2–3 pears of choice, fresh-squeezed juice if required)

Pineapple — Strawberry
(½–1 fresh pineapple or juice from the Skinless Alligator method of "Cutting and Serving Pineapple" as described later in the recipe section, ½–1 cup (118–237 ml) of strawberries, fresh-squeezed juice of preference or distilled water if needed)

Extra Special Shakes

Tropical Delight
Blend 1 papaya, 3–4 bananas, and 1 mango with distilled water to preferred consistency.

Carob Supreme
Blend 3–4 bananas, 4–8 pitted dates, 2–4 de-stemmed black mission figs, 1–2 heaping tablespoons of raw carob powder, and distilled water to reach the desired consistency.

Coconut — Banana Cream
Blend young coconut milk or coconut juice (see *Coconut* in the *Fruit Guide*) with 3–5 bananas, and if needed, just enough distilled water to allow for easy blending.

Sweet Almond
Blend 8–14 almonds (presoaked for easier blending) with 1½ to 2 cups (355–473 ml) of distilled water until the blender runs smoothly for about one minute. Slowly add 3–5 bananas and 4–7 fresh or presoaked pitted dates, along with extra water to desired consistency. *Use any favorite nut or seed for this recipe.*

Tropical Blend
Blend fresh-squeezed orange juice with desired amounts of papaya and one half of a fresh pineapple or the juice from the Skinless Alligator method of "Cutting and Serving Pineapple" as described later in the recipe section.

Juicy Melon
Blend honeydew, cantaloupe, or other melons alone or together to create a *refreshing* light meal.

Fruit Pops

freshly squeezed juice

or

puréed fruits

or

your favorite shake recipe

Commercially sold popsicles are laced with refined sugars, preservatives, and additives, including those enticing and highly hazardous food colors. Instead of opting for store-bought popsicles, why not spend a few minutes to prepare some safe alternatives.

Simply fill popsicle trays with freshly squeezed juices, puréed fruits, or your favorite **Shakes**—thousands of possibilities. See the recipes introduction for advice regarding cold foods.

✎ To prevent fermentation, use cold fruits or shakes and freeze them immediately.

Banana Pops

fully ripe bananas

Bananas make for perfect, quick and easy popsicles. Simply place unpeeled, fully ripe (well-speckled) bananas into resealable freezer bags, set them on baking sheets, and freeze. To eat: thaw until the skin can be easily peeled (bit by bit as you eat) from the *non-stem* end. To prevent freezing your fingers, wrap a cloth around the stem. *Reserve for a hot day!*

✎ Thawing bananas in a bowl of warm water works very well. For *Pops*, thaw them just long enough to loosen the peel so that the stringy parts do not stick to the pulp. If you prefer ice cream or pudding, leave them in the water longer. *Eat immediately.*

Fruit Puddings, Soups, and Sauces

fresh or frozen fruits

freshly squeezed juice or distilled water

dried fruit, unsweetened coconut, raw nuts or seeds (optional)

Blend fresh or frozen fruits, alone, or with small amounts of freshly squeezed juice or distilled water until a pudding, soup, or sauce consistency is reached. Try bananas, pears, apples, stone fruits, berries or any other favorites—*many options! Apple or Apple–Pear Sauce* will get you started.

Those who wish to experiment with exotic flavors should try the following puddings: **Banana–Mango**, **Banana–Persimmon**, **Banana–Berry**, and **Mango–Berry**.

Fill dessert cups or decorative glass bowls with puddings, soups, or sauces, and top with raisins, dried fruits, chopped or whole nuts, coconut, berries, or fruit wedges. *Serve immediately or chill briefly.*

Jams

With a little creativity, it is easy to prepare fresh, delicious jams that are free from refined sugars, additives, and preservatives. Jams are most nourishing and flavorful when freshly prepared, but can be transferred into jars and refrigerated for two or three days. Do not let the following suggestions limit you.

Fig, Date, Raisin Jam

figs, dates, or raisins

distilled water

other dried fruits (optional)

Due to their jelled and seedy consistency, partially rehydrated dried figs can be processed into the perfect jam. Be sure to remove the stems before homogenizing or blending the fruit. Place figs (amount to correspond with the number to be served) in a glass or bowl, pour in enough distilled water to cover by 1 inch (2.5 cm), and soak the fruit until soft enough to allow for easy processing in either your blender or Champion juicer. Blender users should use just enough of the soak water (if fruit is untreated) to move the blades.

Add small amounts of dates or raisins if you wish.

See *Fudge* for *Carob Jam*.

Strawberry (berry) — Pineapple Jam

strawberries (berries)
dried pineapple
distilled water

Simply process soaked, dried pineapple through a Champion Juicer (or with a blender as above) along with fresh or frozen strawberries. For a chunky texture, mix or mash the berries into the processed pineapple. Experiment with different quantities of ingredients to suit your own taste, and the number of people to be served.

Orange — Pineapple Jam

oranges (preferred citrus fruit)
dried pineapple
kiwi (optional)
distilled water

Follow the directions given for strawberry–pineapple jam, and substitute fresh citrus in place of the berries. Truly, these jams can be made to cater to your own tastes, so feel free to add kiwi or other suitable fresh or dried fruits.

Toppings

fresh, frozen, or dried fruits
freshly squeezed juice or distilled water

Prepare delicious, colorful fruit toppings by blending or processing any fruit or combination of fruits with a small amount of freshly squeezed juice or distilled water. Start with **banana–peach** or **mango–raspberry**. Pour toppings over **Fruit Medleys, Ice Creams**, or use as dips for banana slices, strawberries, or fruit wedges. **Jams** make superb toppings with or without the addition of water. See **Fudge** for **Carob Topping**.

Fruit Medleys

acid and sub-acid fruits and/or melons

                              or

sweet, sub-acid, and dried fruits

choice of Topping (optional)

raw nuts or seeds, or coconut (optional)

raw carob powder (optional)

baked oats (optional)

Use a variety of acid and sub-acid fruits, or base the dish on sweet, sub-acid, and dried fruits. Fill a suitable bowl with your favorite fruit wedges, sections, and dried fruits. Fit the serving size to the occasion.

Prepare a *light medley* using oranges, pineapple, strawberries (berries), kiwi, apples, pears, stone fruits, mango, or papaya. Mix the fruits together and serve as is, or drizzle on a complementary **Topping** and dress with unsweetened coconut or raw nuts.

Prepare a *sweet medley* from banana, papaya, mango, pear, or other sweet or sub-acid fruits, and add raisins, dates, figs, or other dried fruits in desired quantities. Garnish to taste.

Classic Medley: 5 bananas, 2 apples, ½ to 1 cup of raisins, and two tablespoons of raw carob powder.

Optional: Those who wish to combine a grain with this dish will find baked oats to be a nice addition. Sprinkle them on top or mix everything together.

Baked Oats

Simply bake oats dry, or use a small amount of distilled water. Dry oats keep longer, but you may prefer the consistency of those that are wetted prior to baking.

Preparation: Pour oats into a large-mouthed bowl and add a *small* amount of distilled water. Mix to lightly wet all the oats (they should not be so wet as to clump together to a great extent) and spread them out on baking sheets. Bake for 8–12 hours at 125–175°F (52-80°C). Place baked oats in glass or plastic containers or airtight freezer bags and store them in the freezer.

Granola

Use plain baked oats as the base for all granola recipes. Simply add your preference of dried fruits, raw nuts or seeds, or raw carob powder to the *pre-baked* oats. Adding the raw ingredients *after* the oats have been cooked gives one the opportunity to obtain every nutrient that the fruits naturally possess. Cooking fruits is contraindicated (see *Raw vs. Cooked* in Part 1).

Ice Creams

Non-fattening, dairy and egg-free ice creams are easy to prepare, and unlike store-bought ice creams, do not contain cholesterol, refined sugars, additives, preservatives, or other chemicals—and they are delicious!

☠ Most commercial ice creams are truly synthetic and hazardous. They have been "created" to be cheap, eye-appealing, and slow-to-melt. Over seventy-five additives (including colors and flavors) are commonly used in commercially sold ice creams. Many of these are among the most harmful. As we examine some of the chemicals that end up in ice creams, keep in mind that children (who happen to be developing brains and nervous systems) compose the largest percentage of victims.

Propylene Glycol Alginate is used as an emulsifier to replace eggs. Eliminating the eggs is beneficial, but this cheap chemical compound is the very same one used in *antifreeze* and *solvents!* Hazards include central nervous system disorders, kidney damage, and birth defects.

Sodium Carbonate, Sodium Hydroxide, and Potassium Hydroxide. These pH-adjusting and water-correcting agents are all highly corrosive. They can cause vomiting, circulatory collapse, and even death!

Calcium Oxide is a pH-adjuster that is also used in fungicides, insecticides, bricks, mortar, and stucco, and for dehairing hides. It is caustic and can severely damage the mucous membranes.

Carrageenan is a thickening agent that has been linked to genetic alterations.

Lactic Acid is a caustic pH-adjuster that can cause vomiting, diarrhea, and gastrointestinal disturbances.

Mono–and Diglycerides are used as emulsifiers. Risks include genetic damage, cancer, and birth defects.

Artificial Colors and Flavors represent the greatest dangers, and the law does not require these to be individually labeled on the packaging. The colors include ***Allura Red*** (could cause cancer and birth defects), ***Amaranth*** and ***Carbon Black*** (carcinogens—both banned in the United States), ***Tartrazine*** (particularly dangerous to those with allergies and asthma, and to those who take acetylsalicylic acid), and ***Fast Green FCF, Paprika***, and ***Brilliant Blue FCF***—all linked to tumor formation.

Flavors used may include *Aldehyde C17* (used in dyes, rubber, and plastic), *Benzyl Acetate* (a solvent), *Butyraldehyde* (used in rubber cement!), *Ethyl Acetate* (a hazardous cleaner for leather and textiles), and *Piperonal* (a lice killer!). Space prohibits further discussion.

> ❏   *The above information was compiled from the following resources: 1995 Encyclopedia of Food Ingredients, A Consumer's Dictionary of Food Additives, The Food Additives Book, Perils of Ice Cream Fact Sheet, Nutrition For Vegetarians, and Emphasis Your Health (Spring 95).*

Salmonella is another potentially lethal hazard found in ice creams—when eggs and dairy products are used. In a single incident in 1994, a well-known ice cream company (distributes throughout the United States) sold salmonella-contaminated products to an unsuspecting public. A total of 2 014 persons reported their illnesses to just one state health department[1]—unsettling, especially when you consider the number of cases that went unreported in this instance, not to mention the countless other poisonings that occur every year.

Obviously, commercially sold ice creams leave little to be desired.

All-Natural Ice Cream

choice of frozen fruit

Bananas, mangos, peaches, nectarines, persimmons, papayas, berries, and fruits with similar consistencies work well for ice creams. Banana and mango ice creams are unsurpassed. Sherbets and ices are made with the frozen forms of juicier fruits.

Simply run frozen fruits through a Champion juicer, or process them with a blender or food processor, adding small amounts of distilled water as needed. To freeze fruits, see the instructions given under each fruit in the *Fruit Guide*.

Carob Ice Cream

frozen, processed bananas

raw carob powder

Simply stir raw carob powder into banana ice cream. Start with a small amount and add more to suit your taste.

Old-Fashioned Ice Cream

frozen bananas or preferred fruits (basic Ice Cream)

dried fruit bits (optional)

raw nuts, seeds, or coconut (optional)

raw carob powder (optional)

fresh fruit (optional)

Mix your choice of dried fruits, chopped nuts, seeds, unsweetened coconut, raw carob powder, preferred berries, or other fruits into banana or another favorite variety of ice cream. *Chewy, chunky, and satisfying!*

Quick'n Easy Ice Cream

choice of frozen fruit

dried fruit bits (optional)

raw nuts or seeds or coconut (optional)

raw carob powder (optional)

fresh fruit (optional)

Quick'n Easy ice cream can be made without any kitchen gadgets or power. The other advantages include little cleanup and less oxidation of the fruit. Simply remove a resealable freezer bag of frozen mango (or other fruit) and thaw it in the refrigerator for several hours until pliable. Leaving the fruit in the bag, gently break it into smaller pieces for even thawing, and place it back into the refrigerator until it can be easily kneaded. Without opening the bag (unless to release excess air), gently knead the semi-frozen fruit with your fists or palms until it is creamy. At this point you may add the ingredients required to make Carob (if using frozen bananas) or Old-Fashioned ice cream. Eat immediately and avoid leftovers.

To eat the fruit warm (as a pudding), thaw it in the refrigerator until soft. Then set the bag into a bowl of warm water and knead gently. Eat *immediately* and do not leave leftovers.

✎ Those who use the Quick'n Easy method should pre-freeze fruits in desired portions. Keep in mind that bananas thaw very quickly.

Ice Cream Parfait

banana or preferred Ice Cream

your favorite Jam

nuts: whole, chopped, or as butter (optional)

unsweetened coconut (optional)

cherries, strawberries, or preferred berry (optional)

Prepare banana or a variety of ice creams and layer them into clear parfait glasses along with **Jams** and raw nuts (whole, chopped, or as butter). If you wish, add whole cherries, strawberries, or preferred berries along the way. Sprinkle with unsweetened coconut and top with a cherry or strawberry.

Super Banana Split

banana or preferred Ice Cream

1 or 2 fresh, fully ripe bananas

your favorite Jam or Topping

fresh fruit sections and wedges, or berries (optional)

unsweetened coconut or raw, chopped nuts (optional)

Peel two bananas and place them opposite each other in a suitable serving dish. If you prefer to use just one banana, then halve it lengthwise. Prepare banana ice cream or even three different varieties if so desired. Spoon three mounds of ice cream between the fresh bananas and top with cherries, berries, or fruit wedges, and your favorite **Jam(s)**. Blend **Jam(s)** with distilled water to create thinner **Toppings** which give a drizzled appearance (see **Toppings** for more alternatives).

Optional: Sprinkle with unsweetened coconut or chopped raw nuts.

Candy

dates (pitted)

figs (de-stemmed)

raisins

distilled water

raw carob powder (optional)

chopped nuts (optional)

raw, unsweetened coconut (optional)

This all-natural candy is satisfying and nutritious. Serve the following recipes moist, firm, or semi-frozen. Experiment with combinations and consistencies until you develop the perfect candy.

Method #1
You need a Champion juicer for this method.

Homogenize (process) one or any combination of the following presoaked fruits: pitted dates, de-stemmed figs, or raisins (in amounts corresponding to the number to be served). Super-soft dates do not require presoaking but should be rinsed. Figs and raisins should be soaked until slightly soft. If you decide to use all three types of fruit, put a little of each into the chute consecutively, so that the combined mass will be thoroughly mixed. The fruit mixture will be sticky to firm depending upon the amount of water that has been absorbed by the fruit during soaking. To keep the mixture dry enough and to prevent loss of sugar, be sure that you only soak the fruit long enough to allow for smooth transport through the appliance.

Form balls or logs from the fruit mass, and roll them in your choice of unsweetened coconut, chopped raw nuts, or raw carob powder. Serve soft, chilled, or freeze on trays and transfer to containers or freezer bags for future use.

Method #2
Use a food processor or blender to work the soaked dried fruits into a sticky mass. Continue as in Method #1.

Method #3
Soak a desired amount of figs, dates, and/or raisins in distilled water until they are just soft enough to be thoroughly mashed together with an appropriate hand tool. Continue as in Method #1.

Fudge

dates (2 parts)

Black Mission figs (1 part)

raisins (1 part)

raw carob powder to taste (optional)

distilled water

chopped nuts (optional)

unsweetened coconut (optional)

Use two parts of dates to single parts of figs and raisins respectively (corresponding to the number of people to be served), and place the ingredients into separate glasses, pouring in enough distilled water to cover the fruit by one inch. Soak the fruits in the refrigerator or at room temperature until soft. Dates and figs that are extremely fresh only need a few minutes of presoaking. Even those that do not require presoaking should be washed to remove dirt. Raisins should be presoaked to enable easy processing and to reveal those that are unfit for consumption. Dates may be pitted and figs de-stemmed prior to soaking.

Process the fruits using your preferred method of making *Candy* (Champion juicer, food processor, blender, or by hand). Hand mix the carob into the fruit mass, adding soak water from the dried fruits as needed. At this point, chopped nuts or unsweetened coconut may be stirred into the mixture (or save and sprinkle on top later). Spread the fudge into a pan and eat immediately, or chill or freeze before serving. Fudge can also be enjoyed as a *Jam* (best with a greater proportion of figs).

Carob Icing, Dip, or Topping
Simply add a little extra water to the fudge recipe to create a creamy carob icing or a dip that is perfect for banana slices, strawberries, or fruit wedges. Adding a bit more water results in a topping.

Banana Logs

Version 1

fresh, fully ripe bananas

your favorite Jam, or Fudge

raw nuts or seeds (optional)

unsweetened coconut (optional)

whole wheat or whole grain bread (optional)

Peel bananas and smother them with your favorite *Jam*. Top with coconut or chopped nuts. Eat immediately, chill briefly, or freeze if necessary. Prepare Carob Logs by spreading on *Icing (see Fudge)*, and if desired, decorate with coconut or chopped nuts.

Optional: Those who wish to combine a grain with either of the Banana Log recipes can wrap whole wheat pita breads or whole grain slices (toasted just enough to remain pliable) around the logs; or better yet, toast the bread until crisp before topping with sliced logs.

📁 Breads should be sweet, light, and thoroughly baked to destroy as many of the yeast germs as possible.[2] In the intestine, live yeast is responsible for robbing the body of B vitamins.[3] B vitamins are vital for liver, kidney, and heart health, the nervous system, and for a number of other organs, glands, and processes. Well-toasting *(but avoid burning)* pre-baked bread will kill the yeast.

Version 2

fresh, fully ripe bananas

nut, seed, or peanut butter

choice of raisins or chopped dates or figs (optional)

whole wheat or whole grain bread (optional)

Peel bananas and spread on a moderate amount of nut, seed, or peanut butter. Top with preferred dried fruit.

Cookies

choice of raisins, dates, or figs

fresh banana (optional)

raw nuts or seeds (optional)

unsweetened coconut (optional)

raw carob powder (optional)

Prepare a desired amount of **Candy** (must be firm), and shape the dried fruit mixture into patties of preferred size. Top with banana slices and your choice of raw carob powder, unsweetened coconut, or raw nuts.

Pies

choice of dates, figs, and/or raisins [approximately 1 lb. (454 g)]

banana or preferred ice cream

fresh or dried fruits (optional)

raw nuts (optional)

unsweetened coconut (optional)

raw carob powder (optional)

Crust

Prepare approximately one pound (454 g) of **Candy** using one or a combination of the following: fresh or dried dates (soaked and pitted); Black Mission, Calimyrna, or Adriatic figs (soaked and de-stemmed), or raisins (soaked). Mold the sticky to slightly firm fruit mass into a pie plate, forming a crust, including the edges. If you wish, make extra for a topping. Place the shell in the freezer to set, and then make the filling.

Filling

Prepare banana or another favorite **Ice Cream** (or even blend two varieties together), and spoon it into the semi-frozen or frozen shell. If you want a layered look, make two varieties of ice cream and layer them in the shell. Decorate with your choice of fruit wedges (peaches, etc.), banana slices, berries, raisins, or raw nuts.

Optional: Sprinkle with unsweetened coconut.

Cover the pie with cellophane and plastic bags, and freeze. Thaw it in the refrigerator just long enough to allow for safe and easy slicing. *For better flavor and more nutrients, put all fresh fruit toppings on immediately before serving.*

Carob Pie
Simply stir raw carob powder into banana ice cream before filling the shell. Garnish with your choice of dried fruits, raw nuts, or unsweetened coconut.

Tropical Pie
Stir unsweetened coconut into banana ice cream and fill your pie shell. Freeze. Thaw slightly, and top with fresh pineapple immediately before serving.

❑   There are many possibilities for pies, so experiment to suit your own tastes.

Papaya Boats

papaya

choice of berries, grapes, melon balls, and fruit wedges

Prepare papaya boats immediately before serving. Halve a papaya and scrape out the seeds. Fill each half with an assortment of your favorite berries, grapes, melon balls, or fruit wedges, and if you wish, serve with a *Pudding* for dipping, or drizzle on a *Topping.*

Milks

It is easy to prepare a variety of quick, nutritious fruit and nut milks, and at the same time avoid the hazards associated with commercially sold cow milk (see Part 1). Changing to nondairy milks is a positive step in the right direction. If you shop wisely, nut milks are even cheaper than cow's milk. *Infants need mother's milk!*

🗁 Keep in mind that these milks are equivalent to the foods themselves, and should therefore be "eaten" (and not simply swallowed), so that the necessary digestive secretions can be released and mixed with the food. Failure to do this will result in incomplete digestion, fermentation or putrefaction, and poisoned blood.

Banana or Fruit Milk

fully ripe bananas or preferred fruits (fresh or frozen)

distilled water

soaked dried fruits (optional)

Follow the directions for making a banana shake (as described earlier in the recipe section), but use less fruit or extra water to taste. To create *a sweeter milk*, blend in a few fresh or soaked dates (pitted), raisins, or figs (de-stemmed). You can easily transform any of your favorite fruits into milks.

🖊 Prepare fruit milks immediately before serving, and do not leave leftovers because processed fruits oxidize and ferment very quickly.

Carob Milk

fully ripe bananas

distilled water

raw carob powder

soaked dried fruits (optional)

Carob milk is the perfect replacement for commercially sold chocolate milk. To find out why, refer to *Carob* and *Cacao* in the *Fruit Guide*, *Factory Farmed Animals and Disease Transmission*, and *Food Combining Principles Tip #1 (Sugars and Milk)* in Part 1.

Preparation: Simply make banana milk as described above and add raw carob powder to taste. For more sweetness, blend in some soft or presoaked dates (pitted), figs (de-stemmed), or raisins.

Nut or Seed Milks

raw, soaked nuts or seeds

distilled water

dates, raisins, or figs (optional)

Blend ¼ cup (59 ml) of cashews, blanched almonds, or any other nuts or seeds with 1 to 1½ cups (237–355 ml) of distilled water until the blender has run calmly for at least 1 to 2 minutes (reduces the amount of pulp). Pour through a sieve or cheesecloth for a smoother texture. Use moderately because nut milks are high in protein.

Nut milks are best fresh, but leftovers can be poured into a tightly sealed container and refrigerated until the following day if necessary.

✐ To allow for easier blending, soak nuts and seeds in a glass of distilled water (or your measuring cup) for a few hours at room temperature or overnight in the refrigerator. Avoid using the soak water because it will contain dirt and undesirable residues. If you do not have time to presoak the nuts, then wash them thoroughly before starting.

For a *sweeter nut milk*, blend in some fresh or soaked pitted dates, de-stemmed figs, or raisins.

Nut or Seed Butters

raw nuts or seeds

distilled water (blender users)

cold pressed oil (for non-oily varieties)

Nut butters make great dips and spreads, and can easily replace every type of fat-saturated spread sold by supermarkets (see *Nuts and Seeds* in the *Fruit Guide* for health research).

Consuming nuts in a butter form does not represent the ideal—whole nuts—but nut butters do have the benefits of versatility and convenience.

If you prefer to buy nut butters then locate a health food store that keeps them refrigerated and has a high turnover rate.

Use a Champion Juicer, grinder, or even a blender for preparing your own nut butters. Process nuts in small quantities to prevent the need for extended storage (less nutrient loss and oxidation) and to avoid overworking the appliance. Always use raw nuts and choose oilier varieties if you prefer to avoid the use of oils. Less oily varieties will require small amounts of oil or distilled water in processing to prevent damage to the appliance and to impart the desired adhesive properties. If you use oil, cold-pressed additive-free types of the same variety as the nuts or seeds that are to be processed are recommended.

Grinders work well, blender users need to combine their nuts with small amounts of distilled water in order to impart the desired cohesive properties. The water reduces the shelf life so these should be consumed within two days. Transfer nut butters into airtight jars and store them in the refrigerator. *Eat moderately!*

Nut, Seed, or Peanut Plums

nut, seed, or peanut butter (sugar, additive, and preservative-free)

prune plums

Gently but thoroughly wash a preferred number of plums. Halve the plums with a sharp knife and then remove the stones (pits). Place a spoonful of nut, seed, or peanut butter on every second half and then rejoin the halves.

✐ Plums bruise very easily and quickly, so be sure to do the preparations immediately before serving.

Melon Boats

watermelon, honeydew, cantaloupe, or preferred melon

grapes, orange sections, or other juicy fruits (optional)

fresh-squeezed lemon or orange juice (optional)

Beautiful, nutritious and delicious melon boats are great for special occasions and large gatherings. Watermelons, honeydews, cantaloupes, or any of other favorite varieties may be used. Make melon boats in sizes that correspond to the occasion, and immediately before serving to prevent oxidation and subsequent nutrient and flavor loss—leftovers are much better as one large chunk of melon rather than in balls and wedges. Cover leftover halves with cellophane and use within two days.

Preparation: Halve or cut melons into desired sizes and scrape out the seeds (remove watermelon seeds when scooping out the balls). Use a melon scoop and spoon out the flesh in balls, quickly placing them into an extra large bowl—or better yet, remove the flesh in chunks. At this time, to increase eye appeal, you may make jagged cuts around the top edge of the melon. Transfer the melon balls (or chunks) into the hull (rind). If you wish, decorate with fruit wedges or sections. Choose juicy, quick-to-digest fruits such as citrus, grapes, mango, or papaya. Freshly squeezed lemon or orange juice will help prevent oxidation. *A colorful cornucopia of succulent fruit!*

"Porcupine" Mango

fully ripe mango

Ripen a mango and use a small, high quality serrated knife to slice down both sides of the pit (from the center on each side of the stem). Hold one half in your palm and make three or four diagonal cuts, being careful not to slice through the skin. Rotate the fruit and make several cuts in the opposite direction to create a checkerboard design. Invert the mango to bring up the "quills." Prepare the second half and serve with the remaining edges.

Cutting and Serving Pineapple

There are three basic methods to prepare pineapple. You need a large, high quality serrated knife. A curved pineapple knife is helpful but not essential. Use a cutting board with a juice border to collect the delicious juice, and to prevent insect problems and the need for extra cleanup.

Boat

1 ripe pineapple

choice of berries, citrus, kiwi, grapes, mango, or papaya (optional)

unsweetened coconut or raw nuts (optional)

preferred Topping or Pudding (optional)

The *Boat* uses the entire fruit except the core, and perhaps the crown if you see fit. Wash the pineapple with warm water and produce soap. Decide whether you want to keep the crown (to remove, twist off) and then slice the fruit in half lengthwise. Use a knife (curved if you have one) to remove the flesh from each half (in quarters if possible). Be careful not to puncture the rind. Chop off the core and cut the flesh into bit-sized chunks, before transferring them back into the two rinds along with any juice. Eat directly from the "boats" or use them as main serving dishes.

Optional: Add color and variety by mixing the pineapple chunks with complementary fruits (1 to 3 varieties) such as strawberries, citrus sections, berries, kiwi, cherries, grapes, mango, or papaya. If you wish, cover with a *Pudding* or *Topping* and decorate with unsweetened coconut or raw nuts.

✐ Whenever possible, prepare all pineapple dishes immediately before serving, and in all other cases, baste with fresh lemon juice, cover tightly in plastic, and refrigerate—even with this treatment, avoid preparations that are more than two hours in advance.

Alligator

1 ripe pineapple

choice of strawberries, citrus, kiwi, mango, or papaya (optional)

unsweetened coconut or raw nuts (optional)

preferred Topping or Pudding (optional)

The *Alligator* is quick and very eye-appealing. Wash the pineapple with warm water and fruit soap. Twist off the crown, chop off the ends, and slice it into lengthwise quarters. Cut the flesh away from each quarter (in one piece) and keep each of the shells. Core and slice each quarter into 10 or 12 chunks before returning them to the shells. Poke the first chunk slightly to one side and the second to the opposite side. Alternate this procedure until you have created four eye-appealing "alligators." Serve alone or complement with your choice of strawberries, citrus sections, kiwi, mango, papaya, raw nuts, or unsweetened coconut. Prepare a *Pudding* for dipping (using forks), or drizzle on a *Topping.*

Skinless Alligator

1 ripe pineapple

choice of berries, citrus, kiwi, grapes, mango, or papaya (optional)

unsweetened coconut or raw nuts (optional)

preferred Topping or Pudding (optional)

This is the most economical way to prepare pineapple because it yields 8–12 ounces of deliciously sweet juice along with the same amount of whole fruit provided by the previous two methods. Follow the instructions for the *Alligator* method until the final step, *or* twist off the crown and chop off both ends, *saving* them for juice. Place the pineapple onto a cutting board (base-side-down). Use a sharp knife to slice away 5 or 6 pieces of shell (lengthwise and keep them) so that you are left with a cylindrical mound of flesh. Hand squeeze the juice from the sections of shell (including the top and bottom) into a large mouthed glass or bowl. Chop the flesh into quarters and core each. Slice the quarters into chunks and serve according to the *Alligator* method except on a plate or platter. Enjoy the juice as is, or use it in your favorite shake recipes.

Salad Dressings

choice of: tomatoes, tomatillos, sweet peppers, cucumbers, celery, zucchini,
broccoli, cauliflower, lemon, avocado, raw nuts, seeds, or olives

distilled water as needed

Use your blender and a combination of vegetables and vegetable-fruits to prepare a wide variety of quick, delicious, and health-friendly dressings. These dressings are free from cholesterol, additives, preservatives, sugars, irritating spices, and vinegars. Allow your taste buds time to become accustomed to these new flavors. Use extra celery (high in organic sodium), green pepper, or tomatillos (see *Tomato*) to add more flavor to those dressings that seem bland at first—your sense of taste may need some restoration. If you use olives, find a safe source and rinse them well. Experiment with different combinations and amounts of ingredients until you have developed some favorites. To preserve the delicate flavors and to enable efficient digestion: keep dressings simple. Use cucumber, juice, or distilled water to make thinner dressings. Soak nuts and seeds briefly to make them softer and to clean off dirt and undesirable residues—dispose of the soak water. Use raw nuts and seeds.

❑   *To reduce oxidation and nutrient loss, dressings should be prepared immediately before serving. Leftovers are not recommended.*

Tomato — Pepper
(try 2–3 large tomatoes with 1 red or green pepper)

Tomato — Avocado
(2–4 tomatoes, 1 avocado)

Tomato — Pepper — Avocado
(3 tomatoes, 1 sweet pepper, and 1 avocado)

Tomato — Celery
(2–4 tomatoes, 2–4 sticks of celery)

Tomato — Celery — Avocado
(2–4 tomatoes, 3–4 celery sticks, and 1 avocado)

Tomato — Nut or Seed — Lemon
(3–5 tomatoes, 2–3 ounces of raw nuts, distilled water. Optional: freshly squeezed lemon juice)

Tomato — Nut or Seed — Pepper or Celery
(3–5 tomatoes, 2–3 ounces of raw nuts, distilled water, pepper or celery to season)

Tomato — Olive
(2–5 tomatoes, 8–16 soaked and rinsed, untreated olives)

Pepper — Cucumber — Celery?
(1 Long-English cucumber, 1 sweet pepper. Optional: celery)

Pepper — Cucumber — Avocado — Celery?
(1 sweet pepper, ½–1 cucumber, 1 avocado. Optional: celery)

Cashew — Orange, Pineapple or Tomato Juice
(2–4 ounces of raw cashews, and freshly squeezed juice to taste)

Vegetable — Avocado — Water
(broccoli or cauliflower, 1 avocado, and distilled water as required)

Salsas and Dips

choice of: tomatoes, tomatillos, bell (sweet) peppers, cucumbers, celery, zucchini, broccoli, cauliflower, fresh lemon, avocado, raw nuts or seeds, or olives

Use the following recipes as dips or toppings for vegetables, grains, and any of your favorite dishes. Prepare a heavier, creamier salsa or dip by blending in avocado. Use any salad dressing recipe for a salsa or dip by simply changing the method of blending. *Chop* or *blend* in spurts so that the vegetable-fruits remain chunky, or mix later with diced vegetables such as celery, pepper, cucumber, tomatoes, tomatillos, and broccoli. For tangy-tart flavor, use tomatillos (see *Tomato*).

Blended Tomatoes
mixed with chopped
Celery, Sweet Pepper, Tomatoes

Blended Tomatoes
mixed with chopped
Celery, Sweet Pepper, Cucumber

Blended Tomatoes
mixed with chopped
Celery, Sweet Pepper, Zucchini

Blended Sweet Pepper and Cucumber
mixed with chopped
Celery

Guacamole
Simply mash ripe avocado by hand. Prepare immediately before serving.

Guacamole Special
Mash 1 large or $1\frac{1}{2}$ small avocados and mix in 1 to 3 sticks of chopped celery. *Optional:* fresh lemon juice or tomatillos. Prepare immediately before serving.

Guacamole Supreme

Mash 1 to 2 large or 2 to 3 small avocados. Dice one stick of celery and one half of a sweet pepper. Blend or chop one or two tomatoes or tomatillos, and mix all of the ingredients together. Prepare immediately before serving.

Stuffed Peppers and Tomatoes

choice of bell (sweet) peppers and tomatoes

preferred guacamole

garnishings (optional)

Wash one or more sweet peppers (any type) thoroughly with produce soap and warm water, and slice the upper third portion off the top of each one. Remove the seeds. You can save the top portions for lids, or dice them and add to your favorite guacamole. Fill the peppers with guacamole and garnish appropriately. Prepare tomatoes in a similar manner.

Center stuffed peppers or tomatoes on platters with crisp vegetables or your favorite dipping foods, or simply serve them alongside any main dish. *Colorful and delicious!*

Eggplant Roll-ups

Japanese eggplants

romaine lettuce

preferred guacamole

tomatoes (optional)

sprouts (optional)

whole wheat pita bread (optional)

Wash thoroughly and place raw Japanese eggplants into large, clean, romaine lettuce leaves. Top with your favorite *Guacamole,* and add slices of tomato or sprouts if you like. Roll them up and eat out of hand, or secure with toothpicks or corn forks and slice them into bite-size rounds during your meal, or immediately before serving others—because eggplant oxidizes *very* quickly.

Optional: Those who wish to combine a grain with this recipe will find whole wheat pita breads to work very well.

As wraps: Toast pitas just enough so that they remain pliable. Place lettuce, one whole Japanese eggplant, guacamole, and optional ingredients on top. Roll them up.

As stiff rounds: Toast pitas until stiff and place lettuce, chopped eggplant, optional ingredients, and guacamole on top.

Creamy Seven Soup

Uncooked tomato-style soups are easy to make with the aid of a food processor or blender. Prepare these soups immediately before serving to prevent oxidation and nutrient loss. Avoid leftovers. You may use room temperature or slightly cool ingredients.

Version 1

7 tomatoes

7 sticks of celery

7 cm (about 3 inches) of cucumber

avocado

pepper (optional)

Blend or process half the tomatoes. Add half the avocado, and half of the remaining ingredients. Work briefly to create a chunky soup or thoroughly for a smooth consistency. Add distilled water as needed. Process the second half of the ingredients and either combine the finished products into one large bowl or pour the soup directly into serving bowls or glasses.

Version 2

7 tomatoes

1½–3 ounces raw cashews or sunflower seeds (presoaked)

celery (to season)

pepper (to season)

Blend or process *(until smooth)* half the tomatoes with half of the nuts or seeds, adding distilled water as needed. Use celery or pepper to season. Pour into a large bowl, smaller bowls, or glasses. Process the remainder of the ingredients.

APPENDIX

<u>TYPICAL STATES OF HEALTH IN WESTERNIZED COUNTRIES</u>

(LISTED FROM HIGHEST TO LOWEST)

Newborn Baby: Generally possesses the highest possible vitality.
- Low toleration level (to poisons and harmful influences)
- Reacts quickly and forcefully when exposed to poisonous matter in an attempt to maintain purity.
- Acute disease symptoms are often extreme, immediate, and violent.

Growing Child: May still have extremely high vitality, depending upon the diet and lifestyle practices instituted by the parents, and whether or not large quantities of drugs were given to suppress disease symptoms (eliminative crises).
- Body will generally tolerate more poisons at this stage.

Young to Middle-aged Adult: Generally has drastically declining vitality due to suppression of disease symptoms.
- Much higher tolerance level is evident.
- Chronic diseases have developed in most.

Elderly (60 plus by today's standards): Generally there is very little vitality left.
- High toleration level.
- Almost all die unnaturally—prematurely due to poor living habits and drug use.
- Chronic diseases are the norm.

ACID AND ALKALINE-FORMING FOODS

ACID FORMING

(DIET SHOULD BE 20%)

*Animal products (flesh, dairy
  products, eggs)
*Legumes (excluding lima beans
  and soybeans)
*Grains (excluding millet)
*Corn (mature)
*Nuts (excluding almonds and
  Coconut)
*Seeds
*Fruits: olives, rhubarb,
  Blueberries, carob, cranberries,
  Currants, plums (including prunes)

ALKALINE FORMING

(DIET SHOULD BE 80%)

*Fruits (nearly all, including
  avocados)
*Non-starchy vegetables (nearly
  all)
*Starchy vegetables (excluding
  mature corn)

Recommended Study

Counsels On Diet And Foods – E. White. Order from ABC at 1-800-765-6955. In California at 1-800-843-8585, and in New York at 1-800-222-3170.

Emphasis Your Health – A Health Journal by Uchee Pines Institute. Order from Uchee Pines Institute, 30 Uchee Pines Road #31, Seale, AL 36875-5702.

Ministry Of Healing – E. White. See *Counsels On Diet And Foods* for ordering information.

The Desire of Ages – E. White. See *Counsels On Diet And Foods* for ordering information.

THE HOLY BIBLE

Scripture Readings

HEALTHFUL LIVING: TODAY, TOMORROW, AND FOR ETERNITY

John 17:3

And this is life eternal, that they might know thee the only true God, and Jesus Christ, whom thou hast sent.

John 10:10

The thief cometh not, but for to steal, and to kill, and to destroy: I am come that they might have life, and that they might have it more abundantly.

3 John 1:2

Beloved, I wish above all things that thou mayest prosper and be in health, even as thy soul prospereth.

Genesis 1:29

And God said, Behold, I have given you every herb bearing seed, which is upon the face of all the earth, and every tree, in the which is the fruit of a tree yielding seed; to you it shall be for meat.

Psalm 141:4

Incline not my heart to any evil thing, to practice wicked works with men that work iniquity: and let me not eat of their dainties.

I Corinthians 6:13

Meats for the belly, and the belly for meats: but God shall destroy both it and them. Now the body is not for fornication, but for the Lord; and the Lord for the body.

Ecclesiastes 10:17

Blessed art thou, O land, when thy king is the son of nobles, and thy princes eat in due season, for strength, and not for drunkenness!

Proverbs 23:1-3

When thou sittest to eat with a ruler, consider diligently what is before thee: And put a knife to thy throat, if thou be a man given to appetite. Be not desirous of his dainties: for they are deceitful meat.

Matthew 4:4

But he answered and said, It is written, Man shall not live by bread alone, but by every word that proceedeth out of the mouth of God.

Micah 4:4

But they shall sit every man under his vine and under his fig tree; and none shall make them afraid: for the mouth of the LORD of hosts hath spoken it.

Isaiah 33:24

And the inhabitant shall not say, I am sick: the people that dwell therein shall be forgiven their iniquity.

Proverbs 23:20–21

Be not among winebibbers; among riotous eaters of flesh: For the drunkard and the glutton shall come to poverty: and drowsiness shall clothe a man with rags.

Proverbs 20:1

Wine is a mocker, strong drink is raging: and whosoever is deceived thereby is not wise.

Proverbs 10:26

As vinegar to the teeth, and as smoke to the eyes, so is the sluggard to them send him.

Psalm 127:2

It is vain for you to rise up early, to sit up late, to eat the bread of sorrows: for so he giveth his beloved sleep.

Ecclesiastes 11:7

Truly the light is sweet, and a pleasant thing it is for the eyes to behold the sun:

Proverbs 3:1–2

My son, forget not my law; but let thine heart keep my commandments: For length of days, and long life, and peace, shall they add to thee.

Psalm 30:2

O LORD my God, I cried unto thee, and thou hast healed me.

Exodus 19:10—11

And the LORD said unto Moses, Go unto the people, and sanctify them today
and tomorrow, and let them wash their clothes, And be ready against the
third day: for the third day the LORD will come down in the sight of the people
upon mount Sinai.

I Corinthians 6:19—20

What? know ye not that your body is the temple of the Holy Ghost which is in
you, which ye have of God, and ye are not your own? For ye are bought with a
price: therefore glorify God in your body, and in your spirit, which are God's.

Proverbs 3:5–8

Trust in the Lord with all thine heart; and lean not unto thine own understanding.
In all thy ways acknowledge him, and he shall direct thy paths. Be not wise in
thine own eyes: fear the Lord, and depart from evil. It shall be health to thy navel,
and marrow to thy bones.

Proverbs 10:27

The fear of the LORD prolongeth days: but the years of the wicked
shall be shortened.

I Corinthians 9:25–27

And every man that striveth for the mastery is temperate in all things. Now they
do it to obtain a corruptible crown; but we an incorruptible. I therefore so run, not
as uncertainly; so fight I, not as one that beateth the air: But I keep under my
body, and bring it into subjection: lest that by any means, when I have preached to
others, I myself should be a castaway.

Proverbs 16:24

Pleasant words are as an honeycomb, sweet to the soul, and health to the bones.

Psalm 103:2–5

Bless the LORD, O my soul, and forget not all his benefits: Who forgiveth all
thine iniquities; who healeth all thy diseases; Who redeemeth thy life from
destruction; who crowneth thee with lovingkindness and tender mercies;
Who satisfieth thy mouth with good things; so that thy youth is renewed
like the eagle's.

Matthew 9:35

And Jesus went about all the cities and villages, teaching in their synagogues, and preaching the gospel of the kingdom, and healing every sickness and every disease among the people.

Romans 12:1–2

I beseech you therefore, brethren, by the mercies of God, that ye present your bodies a living sacrifice, holy, acceptable unto God, which is your reasonable service. And be not conformed to this world: but be ye transformed by the renewing of your mind, that ye may prove what is that good, and acceptable, and perfect will of God.

II Chronicles 16:12

And Asa in the thirty and ninth year of his reign was diseased in his feet, until his disease was exceeding great: yet in his disease he sought not to the LORD, but to the physicians.

Mark 5:25–29

And a certain woman, which had an issue of blood twelve years, And had suffered many things of many physicians, and had spent all that she had, and was nothing bettered, but rather grew worse, When she had heard of Jesus, came in the press behind, and touched his garment. For she said, If I may touch but his clothes, I shall be whole. And straightway the fountain of her blood was dried up; and she felt in her body that she was healed of that plague.

Proverbs 12:10

A righteous man regardeth the life of his beast: but the tender mercies of the wicked are cruel

John 3:14–17

And as Moses lifted up the serpent in the wilderness [see Numbers chapter 21], even so must the Son of man be lifted up: That whosoever believeth in Him should not perish, but have eternal life. For God so loved the world, that he gave his only begotten Son, that whosoever believeth in him should not perish, but have everlasting life. For God sent not his Son into the world to condemn the world; but that the world through him might be saved.

BIBLIOGRAPHY

PART 1

1. Thrash, Agatha, M.D. and Calvin Thrash, M.D., *Nutrition For Vegetarians*. Seale, Alabama: New Lifestyle Books, 1982, pp. 62–67.
2. Vetrano, V. V., B.S., D.C. and Hur, Robin. *The Life Science Health System, Lesson 32*. Austin, Texas: Life Science Institute, 1986, pp. 768–781.
3. Sabitino, Frank, D.C., Ph.D., *Course In Natural Hygiene, Nutrition Part 1, Audio Tape #4*. Huntington, Connecticut: Natural Hygiene Inc. 1985.
4. Khaw, KT. and Barrett-Connor, E. "Dietary Potassium and Stroke Related Mortality." *The New England Journal of Medicine*, 316(5):235–240, January, 1987.
5. Reuben, David, M.D. *Everything You Always Wanted to Know About Nutrition*. New York, New York: Avon Books, 1978, p. 1.
6. Sabitino, Frank, D.C., Ph.D., Natural Hygiene Press Cassette Series. Anemia, Diet, Proteins and Symptoms, Vitamins and Supplements-How they Work, etc., Audio Tape #1. Huntington, Connecticut: Natural Hygiene Inc.
7. Thrash, Agatha, M.D. and Calvin Thrash, M.D., *Nutrition For Vegetarians*. Seale, Alabama: New Lifestyle Books, 1982, p. 69.
8. Thrash, Agatha, M.D. and Calvin Thrash, M.D. *Animal Connection*. Seale, Alabama: New Lifestyle Books, 1983, pp. 43–62.
9. Thrash, Agatha, M.D. and Calvin Thrash, M.D., *Nutrition For Vegetarians*. Seale, Alabama: New Lifestyle Books, 1982, pp. 61–67, 73, 74.
10. Immerman, A., D.C. "Caution: Megavitamins May Be Dangerous To Your Health." *The Life Science Health System, Lesson 9*. Austin, Texas: Life Science Institute, 1986, pp. 240–241.
11. Reuben, David, M.D., *Everything You Always Wanted to Know About Nutrition*. New York, New York: Avon Books, 1978, p. 62.
12. Rothman, KJ, et al. "Teratogenicity of High Vitamin A Intake." *The New England Journal of Medicine*, 333:1369–1373, 1995.
13. *The Lancet*, Vol. 347, February 3, 1996, p. 322.
14. "Vitamin A and Birth Defects." *The New England Journal of Medicine*, 333(21):1414, 1995.
15. Reuben, David, M.D., *Everything You Always Wanted to Know About Nutrition*. New York, New York: Avon Books, 1978, pp. 15–16.
16. Ibid, p. 18
17. Sabitino, Frank, D.C., Ph.D., Natural Hygiene Press Cassette Series. Anemia, Diet, Proteins and Symptoms, Vitamins and Supplements-How they Work, etc., Audio Tape #1. Huntington, Connecticut: Natural Hygiene Inc.
18. Reuben, David, M.D., *Everything You Always Wanted to Know About Nutrition*. New York, New York: Avon Books, 1978, p. 30.
19. Scharffenberg, John, M.D., *Nutrition Update*, Vol. 4, No. 1, pp. 1–2, 1996.
20. Reuben, David, M.D., *Everything You Always Wanted to Know About Nutrition*. New York, New York: Avon Books, 1978, pp. 167–168.

21. Sabitino, Frank, D.C., Ph.D., Natural Hygiene Press Cassette Series. Anemia, Diet, Proteins and Symptoms, Vitamins and Supplements-How they Work, etc., Audio Tape #1. Huntington, Connecticut: Natural Hygiene Inc.

22. Ibid.

23. Foster, Vernon, M.D., *New Start*. Santa Barbara, California: Woodbridge Press 1988, pp. 202–3.

24. Thrash, Agatha, M.D. and Calvin Thrash, M.D., *Nutrition For Vegetarians*. Seale, Alabama: New Lifestyle Books, 1982, pp. 39, 106–107.

25. Benton, Mike. "The Harmfulness of Refined Sugars and Other Sweeteners." *The Life Science Health System, Lesson 30*. Austin, Texas: Life Science Institute, 1986, pp. 715–16.

26. Skorctz, D., *Keys to Health & Happiness*. Loma Linda, California: Reuben A. Hubbard and Daniel Skoretz, 1974.

27. Foster, Vernon, M.D., *New Start*. Santa Barbara, California: Woodbridge Press 1988, p. 203.

28. Thrash, Agatha, M.D. and Calvin Thrash, M.D., *Nutrition For Vegetarians*. Seale, Alabama: New Lifestyle Books, 1982, p. 50.

29. Baldwin, Bernell, Ph.D., *Homeschool Of Health*. Video Presentation: HSOH 011, "Sugar," West Frankfort, Illinois, Three Angels Broadcast Network, 1996.

30. Skoretz, D., "Overfed but Undernourished, Phagocytic Index." *Keys to Health & Happiness*. Loma Linda, California: Reuben A. Hubbard and Daniel Skoretz, 1974.

31. Sanchez, Albert, et al. "Role of Sugars in Human Neutrophilic Phagocytosis." *The American Journal of Clinical Nutrition*, 26:1180–1184, November, 1973.

32. Ibid, pp. 792–94.

33. Allen, Hannah. "Why We Should Not Eat Animal products in Any Form." *The Life Science Health System, Lesson 33*. Austin, Texas: Life Science Institute, 1986, p. 794.

34. Miller, Donald. "Sweetwise." *Emphasis Your Health*. Seale, Alabama: Uchee Pines Institute, Winter, 1995, p. 5.

35. Sanchez, Albert, et al. "Role of Sugars in Human Neutrophilic Phagocytosis." *The American Journal of Clinical Nutrition*, 26:1180–1184, November, 1973.

36. Howe, GR., et al. "Artificial Sweeteners and Human Bladder Cancer." *The Lancet*, 2(8038):578–81, September 17, 1977.

37. Miller, Donald. "Sweetwise." *Emphasis Your Health*. Seale, Alabama: Uchee Pines Institute, Winter, 1995, p. 6.

38. Ibid.

39. Benton, Mike. "The Harmfulness of Refined Sugars and Other Sweeteners." *The Life Science Health System, Lesson 30*. Austin, Texas: Life Science Institute, 1986, p. 719.

40. Porikos, KP, et al. *Physiology & Behavior*, 29(2):293–300, August, 1982.

41. "Paradoxical Effects Of An Intense Sweetener (Aspartame) On Appetite." *The Lancet*, 1092–1093, May 10, 1986.

42. Remington, Dennis, M.D. and Barbara Higa, R.D., *The Bitter Truth About Artificial Sweeteners*. Vitality House, 1987, p. 49.

43. Knighten, Holmes T., *The Journal of the American Dental Association*, Vol. 29, November 1, 1942, pp. 2012–2018.

44. Shelton, Herbert. *The Science and Fine Art of Food and Nutrition*. Oldsmar, Florida: Natural Hygiene Press, 1984, pp. 457–458.
45. Ibid, p. 462.
46. Ibid, p. 463.
47. Skoretz, D., "Overfed but Undernourished." *Keys to Health & Happiness*. Loma Linda, California: Reuben A. Hubbard and Daniel Skoretz, 1974.
48. *American Journal of Physical Anthropology*, 52(4):501–14, May,1980.
49. Shelton, Herbert. *The Science and Fine Art of Food and Nutrition*. Oldsmar, Florida: Natural Hygiene Press, 1984, p. 455.
50. Thrash, Agatha, M.D. and Calvin Thrash, M.D., *Nutrition For Vegetarians*. Seale, Alabama: New Lifestyle Books, 1982, pp. 39, 106–107.
51. Foster, Vernon, M.D., *New Start*. Santa Barbara, California: Woodbridge Press 1988, p. 203.
52. Sanchez, Albert, et al. *The American Journal of Clinical Nutrition*, Vol. 23, No. 6, June 1970, pp. 686–690.
53. Linkosalo, Eeva, et al. *Proc Finn Dent Soc.*, 84:279–86.
54. Ibid.
55. Ibid, p. 283.
56. Miller, C., *Journal Of Nutrition*, Vol. 41, 1950, pp. 70–71.
57. Linkosalo, Eeva, et al. *Proc Finn Dent Soc.*, 1988, 84:253–60.
58. Linkosalo, Eeva, et al. *Proc Finn Dent Soc* 1988, 84, No. 2, p. 113.
59. Millward A., et al. *International Journal of Pediatric Dentistry*, 4(3):151–7, Sept., 1984.
60. Touyz, LZ., *The Journal of the Canadian Dental Association*, 60(5):454–458, May 1994.
61. Shelton, Herbert. *The Science and Fine Art of Food and Nutrition*. Oldsmar, Florida: Natural Hygiene Press, 1984, pp. 464–65.
62. Thrash, Agatha, M.D. and Calvin Thrash, M.D., *Nutrition For Vegetarians*. Seale, Alabama: New Lifestyle Books, 1982, pp. 55–56.
63. Shelton, Herbert. *Superior Nutrition*. San Antonio, Texas: Willow Publishing, Inc., 1987, p. 58.
64. Reuben, David, M.D., *Everything You Always Wanted to Know About Nutrition*. New York, New York: Avon Books, 1978, pp. 153–55.
65. Foster, Vernon, M.D., *New Start*. Santa Barbara, California: Woodbridge Press 1988, p. 206.
66. McDougall, John, M.D., "Weight Control." *Amazing Facts Healthline Series*. Frederick, Maryland: Amazing Facts, 1995, p. 2.
67. Fraser, G. J. Sabat, et al. *Archives of Internal Medicine*, July 1992, Vol. 152, pp. 1416–24.
68. Hardinge, Mervyn, M.D., "Dietary Fatty Acids and Serum Cholesterol Levels." *The American Journal of Clinical Nutrition*, Vol. 10, June 1962, pp. 516–24.
69. Ibid.
70. White, Ellen G., *Counsels On Diet And Foods*. Washington, DC: Review and Herald Publishing Association, 1938, 1946, 1976, p.48.
71. Allen, Hannah. "Why We Should Not Eat Animal products in Any Form." *The Life Science Health System, Lesson 33*. Austin, Texas: Life Science Institute, 1986, p. 801.

72. Foster, Vernon, M.D., *New Start*. Santa Barbara, California: Woodbridge Press 1988, p. 209.

73. Crosby, Neil. *Determination Of Veterinary Residues In Food*. Ellis Horwood Limited, 1991, p. 29.

74. Green, Nancy Sokol. *Poisoning Our Children*. Chicago, Illinois: The Noble Press, 1991, pp. 127–28.

75. Thrash, Agatha, M.D. and Calvin Thrash, M.D., *Animal Connection*. Seale, Alabama: New Lifestyle Books, 1983, pp. 29–36, 67.

76. Green, Nancy Sokol. *Poisoning Our Children*. Chicago, Illinois: The Noble Press, 1991, pp. 127–28, 143.

77. Woolsey, Raymond. *Meat on the Menu: Who Needs It?* Washington, DC: Review and Herald Publishing Association, 1988, pp. 14–15, 24–36.

78. *Realities For The 90's*. Santa Cruz, California: Earthsave Foundation.

79. Robbins, John. *Diet For A New America*. Walpole, New Hampshire: Stillpoint Publishing, 1987, pp. 65, 109, 1177.

80. Allen, Hannah. "Why We Should Not Eat Meat." *The Life Science Health System, Lesson 32*. Austin, Texas: Life Science Institute, 1986, p. 746–47.

81. Thrash, Agatha, M.D. and Calvin Thrash, M.D., *Nutrition For Vegetarians*. Seale, Alabama: New Lifestyle Books, 1982, p. 8.

82. "Going Meatless." *Vibrant Life, A Special Issue On Vegetarianism*. Hagerstown, Maryland: Review and Herald Publishing, 1992, pp. 21, 29.

83. Thrash, Agatha, M.D., *Help Yourself To Health*, video presentation #15: Cancer. West Frankfort, Illinois, Three Angels Broadcast Network, 1996.

84. Ibid.

85. Miller, Donald. "BSE." *Emphasis Your Health*. Seale, Alabama: Uchee Pines Institute, Vol. 12, No. 2, 1995, pp. 11–13.

86. Ibid.

87. Berkelman, R., *The Journal of Infectious Diseases*,170:272–73, August, 1994.

88. Skoretz, D., "Christianity and Health." *Keys to Health & Happiness*. Loma Linda, California: Reuben A. Hubbard and Daniel Skoretz, 1974.

89. Ibid.

90. Ibid.

91. Benton, Mike. "Proteins in the Diet." *The Life Science Health System, Lesson 8*. Austin, Texas: Life Science Institute, 1986, p. 214.

92. *Earthsave*, Spring & Summer 1992, Vol. 3, Numbers 2 & 3, p.26.

93. Feighner, B, et al. *American Journal of Epidemiology*, 136(7):836–42, Oct. 1, 1992.

94. McGeehin, MA, et al. *American Journal of Epidemiology*, 138(7):492–501, Oct. 1, 1993.

95. Morris, RD et al. *American Journal of Public Health*, 82(7):955–63, July, 1992.

96. Koivusalo, M., et al. *American Journal of Public Health*, 84(8):1223–8, August, 1994.

97. Pilotto, LS., *The Australian Journal of Public Health*, 19(1):89–93, February, 1995.

98. Dunnick, JK., RL. Melnick. *Journal of the National Cancer Institute*, 85(10):817–22, May 19, 1993.

99. Keough, Carol. *Water Fit to Drink*. Emmaus, Pennsylvania: Rodale Press, 1980, p. 22.

100. *Edmonton Journal*, Nov. 23, 1995, p. A3.

101. Ibid, Dec. 6, 1995, p. A3.
102. "A Brief Report on the Association of Drinking Water Fluoridation and the Incidence of Osteosarcoma Among Young Males." *New Jersey Department of Health*, November 1992.
103. "Fluoride, the Aging Factor," *Health Action Press*, pp. 72–90, 1993.
104. Null, Gary. *Clearer, Cleaner, Safer, Greener*. New York, Toronto: Random House, 1990, p. 66.
105. "Don't Drink the Water?" *Newsweek*, Feb. 5, 1990.
106. Null, Gary. "The Fluoride Fiasco." Townsend Letter for Doctors & Patients, August–September 1996, pp. 56–65.
107. Jacobsen, SJ., et al. "Hip Fracture Incidence Before and After the Fluoridation of the Public Water Supply..." *American Journal of Public Health*, 83(5):743–5, May, 1993.
108. Jacobsen, SJ., et al. "The Association Between Water Fluoridation and Hip Fracture..." *Annals of Epidemiology*, 2(5):617–26, Sept., 1992.
109. Riordan, PJ. "Dental Fluorosis, Dental Caries and Fluoride Exposure Among 7-year-olds." *Caries Research*, 27(1):71–77, 1993.
110. Freni, SC. "Exposure to High Fluoride Concentrations In Drinking Water Is Associated With Decreased Birth Rates." *Journal of Toxicology & Environmental Health*, 42(1):109–21, May, 1994.
111. Walker, G. "Fluorides and Birth Defects." *The Australian Fluoridation News*, Vol. 31, No. 5, Sept.–Oct. 1995.
112. Li, XS., et al. "Effect of Fluoride Exposure on Intelligence in Children." *Fluoride*, Vol. 28, No. 4, 1995, pp. 189–192.
113. Mullenix, Phyllis J., et al. *Neurotoxicology and Teratology*, Vol. 17, No. 2, pp. 169–177, 1995.
114. Shelton, Herbert. *The Science and Fine Art of Food and Nutrition*. Oldsmar, Florida: Natural Hygiene Press, 1984, p. 400
115. Ibid, p. 403.
116. Ibid, pp.401–402.
117. Ibid, p. 401.
118. Ibid, p. 401.
119. Fry, Marti, and Norman Allard. "The Role of Acid and Alkaline Substances Within the Body." *The Life Science Health System, Lesson 12*. Austin, Texas: Life Science Institute, 1986, pp. 303, 305.
120. Massey, R.C., and M.J. Dennis. *Food Additives And Contaminants*, Vol. 4, No.1, 1987, pp. 27–36.
121. Thrash, Agatha, M.D. and Calvin Thrash, M.D., *Nutrition For Vegetarians*. Seale, Alabama: New Lifestyle Books, 1982, p. 66.
122. Shelton, Herbert. *The Science and Fine Art of Food and Nutrition*. Oldsmar, Florida: Natural Hygiene Press, 1984, p. 330
123. Hardinge, Mervyn, M.D., "The Case For Vegetarianism." *The Journal Of Health & Healing*, Vol. 16, No.1, 1992, pp. 30 and 40.
124. *The Journal Of Health & Healing*. Wildwood, Georgia: Wildwood Lifestyle Center & Hospital, Vol. 16, No.1, 1992, pp. 42–43.

125. Allen, Hannah. "Why We Should Not Eat Meat." *The Life Science Health System, Lesson 32*. Austin, Texas: Life Science Institute, 1986, p. 745.
126. Scharffenberg, John. *The Journal Of Health & Healing*, Vol. 16, No.1, 1992, pp. 20–21.
127. Hardinge, Mervyn, M.D., and Fredrick Stare, M.D., "Nutritional Studies Of Vegetarians." *The Journal Of Clinical Nutrition*, Vol. 2, No. 2, March-April, 1954, pp. 83–88.
128. Scharffenberg, John. *The Journal Of Health & Healing*, Vol. 16, No.1, 1992, pp. 20–21.
129. *Health Science*, Tampa Florida: American Natural Hygiene Society, Vol. 18, No. 1, January–February, 1995, p. 10.
130. Skoretz, D., "Miracle of Hunza - Why They Live Longer." *Keys to Health & Happiness*. Loma Linda, California: Reuben A. Hubbard and Daniel Skoretz, 1974.
131. Hardinge, Mervyn, M.D., and Hulda Crooks. "Non-Flesh Dietaries." Journal Of *The American Dietetic Association*, Vol. 45, No. 6, December, 1964, p. 538.
132. Resnicow, Ken, et al. "Diet and Serum Lipids In Vegan Vegetarians: A Model For Risk Reduction." Journal Of *The American Dietetic Association*, Vol. 91, No.4, April, 1991, pp. 447–53.
133. Shelton, Herbert. *The Science and Fine Art of Food and Nutrition*. Oldsmar, Florida: Natural Hygiene Press, 1984, p. 523.
134. Ibid.
135. Ibid, pp. 523–524.
136. Sloane, Philip D., M.D., and Salli Benedict, M.P.H., and Melanie Mintzer, M.D., *The Complete Pregnancy Workbook*. Toronto, Ontario: Key Porter Books Limited, 1987, p. 190.
137. Ibid.
138. Shelton, Herbert. *The Science and Fine Art of Food and Nutrition*. Oldsmar, Florida: Natural Hygiene Press, 1984, pp. 523–524.
139. Ibid, pp. 558–560
140. Ibid, pp. 539–540
141. McDougall, John, M.D., "Diabetes." *Amazing Facts Healthline Series*. Frederick, Maryland: Amazing Facts, 1995.
142. Ibid.
143. McDougall, John, M.D., "Diabetes." *Amazing Facts Healthline Series*. Frederick, Maryland: Amazing Facts, 1995, p. 3.
144. Thrash, Agatha, M.D., *Emphasis Your Health*. Seale, Alabama: Uchee Pines Institute, Summer–Fall 1993, p. 20.
145. Tremblay, A., et al. *International Journal of Obesity & Related Metabolic Disorders*, 19(2):79–86, Feb., 1995.
146. Goldberg, GR., et al. *European Journal of Clinical Nutrition*, 44(2):99–105, Feb., 1990.
147. Hardinge, Mervyn, M.D., et al. *Life and Health, National Health Journal*. Washington D.C.: Review and Herald Publishing Association, 1973.
148. Watterson, Andrew. *Pesticides and Your Food*. London: The Merlin Press, 1991, p. 3.

149. Mott, L., and K. Snyder. *Pesticide Alert: A Guide to Pesticides in Fruit and Vegetables*. San Francisco, CA: Sierra Club Books, 1987, p. 5.

150. Ibid, p. 7.

151. *Earthsave*, Spring & Summer 1992, Vol. 3, Numbers 2 & 3, p.14.

152. Mott, L., and K. Snyder. *Pesticide Alert: A Guide to pesticides in Fruit and Vegetables*. San Francisco, CA: Sierra Club Books, 1987, p. 7.

153. *Global Pesticide Campaigner*, Vol. 6, No. 2, June, 1996, p. 18. San Francisco, CA: Pesticide Action Network.

154. Keough, Carol. *Water Fit to Drink*. Emmaus, Pennsylvania: Rodale Press, 1980, p. 29.

155. " Action Alert." *Food & Water*. Walden, Vermont, 1996.

156. *Food & Water*. Personal letter from Suzanna Jones, August 13, 1996.

157. *Ca—A Cancer Journal For Clinicians*, Vol. 46, No. 1, January–February, 1996, p. 8.

158. "Pesticides and Their Effect on Children," Reprint from NCAMP's *Safety at Home: A Guide to the Hazards of Lawn and Garden Pesticides*, 1996, p. 63.

159. McCuen, Gary. *Poison In Your Food*. Hudson, Wisconsin: Gary E. McCuen Publications Inc., 1991, p. 60.

160. "Pesticides and Their Effect on Children," Reprint from NCAMP's *Safety at Home: A Guide to the Hazards of Lawn and Garden Pesticides*, 1996, p. 63.

161. Davis, James, Ph.D. "Childhood Brain Cancer Linked To Consumer Pesticide Use." *Pesticides and You*, Spring, 1993, pp. 18–20.

162. *Earthsave*, Spring & Summer 1992, Vol. 3, Numbers 2 & 3, p.14.

163. Lamb, Marjorie. *Two Minutes A Day For A Greener Planet*. Toronto, Ontario: Harper-Collins Publishers Ltd., 1990, p. 184.

164. "Healthy Food and Healthy Farms." *Northwest Coalition for Alternatives to pesticides, Fact Sheet*, December, 1993.

165. Ibid.

166. Moyer, Bill. "In Our Children's Food." *Frontline*, March 30, 1993.

167. Mott, L., and K. Snyder. *Alert: A Guide to Pesticides in Fruit and Vegetables*. San Francisco, CA: Sierra Club Books, 1987, p. 70.

168. "Postharvest Treatments." *Northwest Coalition for Alternatives to Pesticides, Fact Sheet*, December, 1996.

169. Ibid.

170. Mott, L., and K. Snyder. *Alert: A Guide to Pesticides in Fruit and Vegetables*. San Francisco, CA: Sierra Club Books, 1987, p. 126.

171. Green, Nancy Sokol. *Poisoning Our Children*. The Noble Press, 1991, pp. 36–37.

172. Robbins, John. *Diet For A New America*. Walpole, New Hampshire: Stillpoint Publishing, 1987, p. 343.

173. Seager, Joni. *The State Of The Earth Atlas*. Touchstone/Simon and Schuster, 1990, pp. 104–105.

174. Seager, Joni. *The State Of The Earth Atlas*. Touchstone/Simon and Schuster, 1990, pp. 105.

175. *Global Pesticide Campaigner*, Vol. 6, No. 2, June, 1996, pp. 4–5. San Francisco, CA: Pesticide Action Network

176. Seager, Joni. *The State Of The Earth Atlas*. Touchstone/Simon and Schuster, 1990, pp. 104–105.

177. Robbins, John. *Diet For A New America*. Walpole, New Hampshire: Stillpoint Publishing, 1987, p. 343.
178. Scharffenberg, John, M.D., *The Journal Of Health & Healing*. Wildwood, Georgia: Wildwood Lifestyle Center & Hospital, Vol. 16, No.1, 1992, pp. 20–21.
179. Ibid.
180. Robbins, John. *Diet For A New America*. Walpole, New Hampshire: Stillpoint Publishing, 1987, p. 315.
181. Diamond, Harvey. *Your Heart Your Planet*. Santa Monica, CA: Hay House, Inc., 1990, p. 76.
182. Robbins, John. *Diet For A New America*. Walpole, New Hampshire: Stillpoint Publishing, 1987, p. 317.
183. Hergenrather, Jeffrey, et al. *The New England Journal Of Medicine*, March 26, 1981, p. 792.
184. *Pure Food Campaign–Canada Chapter*, Press Releases, June 25th and July 2nd, 1993.
185. Cummins, Joseph. *Alive*, #130, May 1993, pp. 12–13.
186. Bullard, Linda. "Genetic Engineering and Foodstuffs." *European Greens*, 1991. Reprint obtained from Pure Food Campaign, 1993.
187. *Food & Water Journal*, Vol. 5, No. 2, Spring 1996, p. 9. Walden, Verment: Food & Water Inc.
188. Moyer, Bill. "In Our Children's Food." *Frontline,* March 30,1993.
189. *Action Link*, August 1995. Ottawa, Ontario: Action Link.
190. Ibid.
191. "Answers To Questions About BGH." Food & Water Fact Booklet. Walden, Verment: Food & Water Inc., 1996.
192. McCuen, Gary. *Poison In Your Food*. Hudson, Wisconsin: Gary E. McCuen Publications Inc., 1991, p. 60.
193. Ibid.
194. *Fact Sheet On Food Irradiation*. Burnaby, British Columbia: Health Action Network Society, 1993.
195. *Fact Sheet On Food Irradiation*. Burnaby, British Columbia: Health Action Network Society, 1993.
196. Bhaskaram, C., and G. Sadasivan. *The American Journal of Clinical Nutrition*, No. 28, February 1975, pp. 130–135.
197. Leemhorst, J.G., *Food Irradiation Now*. Nijhoff/Junk Publishers, 1982, p. 1.
198. White, E.G., *Ministry of Healing*. Elizabethton, Tennessee: MLI Software, 325. Copy of original work: *Ministry of Healing*. Mountain View, California: Pacific Press Publishing Association,1905.
199. White, E.G., *Christian Temperance and Bible Hygiene*. Elizabethtown, Tennessee: MLI Software, 46. Copy of original work: *Christian Temperance and Bible Hygiene*: Mountain View, California: Pacific Press Publishing Association, 1890.
200. *Earthsave*, Spring & Summer 1992, Vol. 3, Numbers 2 & 3, p. 9.
201. *Realities For The 90's*. Santa Cruz, California: Earthsave Foundation, p. 3.
202. Ibid.
203. Robbins, John. *Diet For A New America*. Walpole, New Hampshire: Stillpoint Publishing, 1987, p. 367.

204. *Realities For The 90's*. Santa Cruz, California: Earthsave Foundation, p. 2.

205. Ibid, p. 3.

206. *Earthsave*, Spring & Summer 1992, Vol. 3, Numbers 2 & 3, p.14.

207. *Realities For The 90's*. Santa Cruz, California: Earthsave Foundation, pp. 5–6.

208. Shelton, Herbert. *Food Combining Made Easy*. San Antonio, Texas: Willow Publishing Inc., 1982, p. 24.

209. Veith, Dr. Walter. "Life At It's Best - Part 1." *Amazing Discoveries Video Presentation*. Delta, B.C.: Amazing Discoveries, 1993.

210. Thrash, Agatha, M.D. and Calvin Thrash, M.D., *Animal Connection*. Seale, Alabama: New Lifestyle Books, 1983, p. 52.

211. White, Ellen G., *Counsels On Diet And Foods*. Washington, DC: Review and Herald Publishing Association, 1938, 1946, 1976, pp. 263–264.

212. *Feeding a Crowd Safely*. Edmonton, Alberta: Alberta Agriculture, Homedex 1123, p. 3.

213. Ibid.

Part 2

1. International Apple Institute. *Apples: A Class Act,* 1995, p. 3.

2. Ibid, p.5.

3. Seelig, R.A., *Bananas*. Alexandria, Virginia: United Fresh Fruit and Vegetable Association, 1995, p. 6.

4. Ibid, p. 4.

5. Ibid, pp. 6–7.

6. Lessard, W.O., *The Complete Book Of Bananas*. W.O. Lessard, 1992, p. 3.

7. Ibid, p. 3.

8. Ibid, p. 5.

9. Seelig, R.A., *Bananas*. Alexandria, Virginia: United Fresh Fruit and Vegetable Association, 1995, p. 33.

10. Lessard, W.O., *The Complete Book Of Bananas*. W.O. Lessard, 1992, p. 47.

11. Ibid, p. 81.

12. North American Blueberry Council. *The Blueberry Bulletin*. Marmora, N.Y.: 1995, p. 2.

13. Ibid.

14. Ibid.

15. Field Enterprises Educational Corporation. *The World Book Encyclopedia*, Vol. 4, Ci to Cz, 1968, p. 953.

16. California Strawberry Advisory Board. *California Srawberries With Style*. Watsonville, California: California Strawberry Advisory Board.

17. Thrash, Agatha, M.D., Calvin Thrash, M.D., Donald Miller. *Poison With A Capital C*. Seale, Alabama: New Lifestyle Books, 1991, pp. 4–14.

18. Ibid, pp. 15–17.

19. Ibid, p. 16.

20. Healthful Living Series, Pamphlet #6.

21. Florida Department Of Citrus. *Florida's True Colors*, 1993, p. 22.

22. Ibid, p. 7.

23. Freydberg, Nicholas, Ph.D., and Willis A. Gortner, Ph.D., *The Food Additives Book*. New York, New York: Bantam Books Inc., 1982, p. 537.
24. Green, Nancy Sokol. *Poisoning Our Children*. The Noble Press, 1991, pp. 130–131.
25. Florida Department Of Citrus. *Guide*, back page.
26. Florida Department Of Citrus. *Florida's True Colors*, 1993, p. 3.
27. Field Enterprises Educational Corporation. *The World Book Encyclopedia, Vol. 5*, D, 1968, pp. 34–35.
28. Down To Earth Natural Foods. *Dates Fact Sheet*, 1994.
29. Esser, William. *Dictionary Of Natural Foods*. Bridgeport, Connecticut: Natural Hygiene Press, 1983, p. 55.
30. Esser, William. *Dictionary Of Natural Foods*. Bridgeport, Connecticut: Natural Hygiene Press, 1983, p. 56.
31. Sharman M., *Food Additives & Contaminants*, 8(3):299–304, 1991, May-June.
32. Oski, Frank, M.D., *Don't Drink Your Milk*. Brushton, New York: TEACH Services, Inc., 1992, p. 48
33. Shelton, Herbert. *The Science and Fine Art of Food and Nutrition*. Oldsmar, Florida: Natural Hygiene Press, 1984, p. 523.
34. Oski, Frank, M.D., *Don't Drink Your Milk*. Brushton, New York: TEACH Services, Inc., 1992, all.
35. Thrash, Agatha, M.D. and Calvin Thrash, M. D., *Animal Connection*. Seale, Alabama: New Lifestyle Books, 1983, Chapters 3–17.
36. California Fig Advisory Board. *Fig News*, p. 6.
37. California Raisin Advisory Board. *California Raisins, A Food Manufacturer's Guide*, Nov. 4, 1993, p. 2.
38. Moyers, Bill. *Frontline: In Our Children's Food*, March 30,1993.
39. Thrash, Agatha, M.D., *Emphasis Your Health*. Seale, Alabama: Uchee Pines Institute, Vol. 13, No. 2, 1997, p. 18.
40. Esser, William. *Dictionary Of Natural Foods*. Bridgeport, Connecticut: Natural Hygiene Press, 1983, p. 68.
41. Redland's Fruit and Spice Park. *Plant Guide*. Homestead, Florida: Redland's Fruit and Spice Park, p. 59.
42. National Watermelon Promotion Board. *Citrulius Lanatus Watermelon*. Orlando, Florida: National Watermelon Promotion Board, p. 6.
43. Heritage, Ford. *Composition and Facts About Foods.*, 1971, p. 43.
44. TLC, *The Learning Channel*. "Jesus and His Times."
45. Field Enterprises Educational Corporation. *The World Book Encyclopedia*, Vol. 14, N-O, 1968, p. 564.
46. Garrido, A., et al. *Nahrung*, 37(6):583–91, 1993.
47. Thrash, Agatha, M.D. and Calvin Thrash, M.D., *Nutrition For Vegetarians*. Seale, Alabama: New Lifestyle Books, 1982, p. 83.
48. Redland's Fruit and Spice Park. *Plant Guide*. Homestead, Florida: Redland's Fruit and Spice Park, p. 58.
49. Ibid.
50. Heritage, Ford. *Composition and Facts About Foods.* , 1971, p. 9.
51. Oregon Washington California Pear Bureau. *The Encyclopedia of Pears*. Portland, Oregon, 1995, p. 1.

52. Field Enterprises Educational Corporation. *The World Book Encyclopedia*, Vol. 15, P, 1968, p. 191.

53. Hessayon, D.G., *The Fruit Expert*. England: pbi Publications,p. 27.

54. Esser, William. *Dictionary Of Natural Foods*. Bridgeport, Connecticut: Natural Hygiene Press, 1983, p. 94.

55. Field Enterprises Educational Corporation. *The World Book Encyclopedia*, Vol. 15, P, 1968, p. 424.

56. Redland's Fruit and Spice Park. *Plant Guide*. Homestead, Florida: Redland's Fruit and Spice Park, p. 24.

57. Field Enterprises Educational Corporation. *The World Book Encyclopedia*, Vol. 17, S, 1968, p. 107.

58. Veith, Dr. Walter. "Life At It's Best - Part 1." *Amazing Discoveries Video Presentation*. Delta, B.C.: Amazing Discoveries, 1993.

59. Thrash, Agatha, M.D. and Calvin Thrash, M.D., *Nutrition For Vegetarians*. Seale, Alabama: New Lifestyle Books, 1982, pp. 49–50.

60. Shelton, Herbert. *The Science and Fine Art of Food and Nutrition*. Oldsmar, Florida: Natural Hygiene Press, 1984, p. 74

61. Stammati A., et al. *Food Additives & Contaminants,* 9(5):551–60, 1992, September–October.

62. Shelton, H.M., *Superior Nutrition*. San Antonio, Texas: Willow Publishing, Inc., 1987, p. 74.

63. Fazio, T. and C. R. Warner. *Food Additives & Contaminants*, Vol. 7, No. 4, 1990, pp. 433–454.

64. Ibid.

65. Stammati A., et al. *Food Additives & Contaminants*, 9(5):551–60, 1992, September–October.

66. Armentia-Alvarez, A., et al. *Food Additives & Contaminants*, 10(2):157–165, 1993, March–April.

67. Til, HP. and VJ. Feron. *Food Additives & Contaminants*, 9(5):587–95, 1992, September–October.

68. California Raisin Advisory Board. *California Raisins, A Food Manufacturer's Guide*, Nov. 4, 1993, p. 2.

69. Ibid.

70. California Raisin Advisory Board. *California Raisins, A Food Manufacturer's Guide*, Nov. 4, 1993, p. 1.

71. California Raisin Advisory Board. "*California Raisins - A Harvest Of Sunshine.*" Fresno, California: California Advisory Board, March 1987, p. 1.

72. California Raisin Advisory Board. "*California Raisins - A Harvest Of Sunshine.*" Fresno, California: California Advisory Board, March 1987.

73. California Raisin Advisory Board. "*California Raisins - A Harvest Of Sunshine.*" Fresno, California: California Advisory Board, March 1987.

74. Ibid

75. Sabaté, Joan, and Gary E. Fraser. "Nuts: A New Protective Food Against Coronary Heart Disease." *Current Opinion in Lipidology*, 1994, 5:11–16.

76. Sabaté, Joan, et al. *Archives of Internal Medicine*, Vol. 152, July, 1992, pp. 1416–24.

77. Thrash, Agatha, M.D. and Calvin Thrash, M.D., *Nutrition For Vegetarians*. Seale, Alabama: New Lifestyle Books, 1982, pp. 82–85.

78. Oski, Frank, M.D., *Don't Drink Your Milk*. Brushton, New York: TEACH Services, Inc., 1992, pp. 48–49.

79. Shelton, Herbert. *The Science and Fine Art of Food and Nutrition*. Oldsmar, Florida: Natural Hygiene Press, 1984, p. 148.

80. "Aflatoxins." *Health Protection Branch Issues*. Ottawa, Ontario: Health Canada, May 1990, p. 2.

81. "Aflatoxins." *Health Protection Branch Issues*. Ottawa, Ontario: Health Canada, May 1990, p. 3.

82. Thrash, Agatha, M.D. and Calvin Thrash, M.D., *Nutrition For Vegetarians*. Seale, Alabama: New Lifestyle Books, 1982, p. 84.

PART 3

1. *JAMA*, Vol. 272, No.19, November 16, 1994, p. 1492
2. White, Ellen G. Estate. *Medical Science and the Spirit of Prophecy*. Washington, DC: Review and Herald Publishing Association, 1971, pp. 10–11.
3. Ibid.

Index

****
NOTES

****

NOTES

****

NOTES

****
NOTES

****

NOTES

****

NOTES

****
NOTES

****

NOTES

****
NOTES

****
NOTES

NOTES

****

NOTES